CONFESSIONS *of an*
UNLIKELY
RUNNER

A Guide to Racing and Obstacle
Courses for the Averagely Fit and
Halfway Dedicated

By Dana Ayers

COPYRIGHT

Cover Design: John Matthews, updates by Amanda Downey

Editing: Grace Kerina

Author photo courtesy of Kami Swingle

Tough Mudder photo courtesy of an unknown photographer. If it's you, please contact the author

Flosser photo courtesy of Dana Ayers

ADVANCE PRAISE

"A must-read for anyone that has ever had a mishap during a race, Dana Ayers' book is a hilarious ride from beginning to end. Whether you're an experienced marathoner or brand new to the sport, you'll appreciate Dana's witty, down-to-earth style as she describes her experiences with mud runs, marathons and everything in between. With tons of pro tips sprinkled throughout, this book has something for everyone, and by the end, even non-runners will want to lace up their shoes and go for a run!"

JILL ANGIE
RRCA-certified running coach and author of *Running With Curves: Why You're Not Too Fat to Run, and the Skinny on How to Start Today*

"While our running experiences differ, Ayers shares my love for the sport of running and the running community. This is a fun read for anyone who is a runner, and motivational for anyone who is not yet a runner. Very entertaining!"

JIM RYUN
Olympic Silver Medalist and Mile Record-Holder

"Dana Ayers shows—by trying marathons, obstacle races, road relays both standard and seat-of-the-pants—that the only barrier for being a runner isn't the speed you move, but your willingness to challenge yourself and try new things. She relates experiences in the sport in a way that makes even the bizarre sound appealing and grounds them all in a way that can draw in even a reluctant runner."

CHARLIE BAN
Editor in Chief, *RunWashington* magazine

"If you've ever made it a goal to finish a marathon or complete a Tough Mudder, read this book. It won't run the race for you, but it will motivate and entertain you, which is probably better. Ayers is like a cross between Mindy Kaling and Bridget Jones, but her stories have at least 75% more thigh-chafing and pants-ripping."

LINDSAY APPLEBAUM
Former Editor, *Sports Illustrated* and *The Washington Post*

"What a totally delightful read! Uplifting, encouraging, funny and inspiring. This is a book I'll be recommending and sharing with many of my friends. As a coach I cringed a little at the description of Ayers' 'limited preparation' for some of her races but at the same time I smiled at her tenacity and marveled at her ability to overcome and complete her goals. Ayers' humility and her adventures made me laugh out loud and at times nod in a shared 'I've been there' sort of way. Thanks for making me smile!"

JANET HAMILTON
Registered Clinical Exercise Physiologist and owner of Running Strong Professional Coaching, www.runningstrong.com

---

"You can't help but laugh and completely relate to Dana Ayers' escapades in her book, *Confessions of an Unlikely Runner*. Unlike Dana, I did grow up as an athlete, and I did run in college—by force, in formation, all while singing cadences at West Point. At that time, being a back of the pack runner was something no one wanted to be. But after many years of not running since leaving college and active duty service, I have re-discovered my running form, this time at the back of the pack. Some of the most inspirational people with the greatest stories reside at the back of the pack. I've experienced incredible joy running along-side them, encouraging them, and using their stories as my motivation. I still don't love running, but, like Dana, I've discovered that we don't necessarily run to compete. We run to be with each other. The best part? Everyone can be a back of the pack runner!"

GEORGINA BIEHL
Regional Director, Team Red, White & Blue — "Enriching the lives of America's veterans through physical and social activity"

"This book is laugh-out-loud-funny and describes experiences that anyone can relate to. Dana Ayers expertly blends stories from her journey as a 'recreational' runner and athlete with a genuine voice filled with humor and humility. This is a must-read for hesitant runners and I hope Ayers writes about more of her adventures soon!"

GINA JUNIO
Mentor, *Team in Training* Endurance Sports Training Program, and Certified Personal Trainer

---

TABLE OF CONTENTS

INTRODUCTION

I round the corner and head back to where my supplies are, glancing down to make sure the tourniquet around my thigh is holding up. I've been fighting for nearly four hours. I notice strangers eyeing me warily, and I press on. This must be exactly how Rambo felt... if he was real, and if he was bandaged up because he'd split the upper inside seam of his yoga pants wide open on mile 13 of a 20-mile run... like I just had.

I'm not fighting in the jungles of Southeast Asia, I'm marathon training. And the gaping hole, dangerously close to revealing my unmentionables, chafes in an unfortunate location.

I'd tell you this is the only embarrassing horror story from my more than ten years of running, but that'd be grossly incorrect. I've tripped. I've come in last. I've watched bubbles cover the sleeves of my jacket during a rainy group run, after my washing machine played a cruel joke and didn't rinse my clothes appropriately. I've freaked out when I met someone's pet snake on a trail. I've vomited during a race. *Twice.* But I'm here to tell you that it's possible to keep going, even when running doesn't come naturally. And I'm here to tell you why it's worth it to keep going in this crazy sport.

I'm what is sometimes lovingly referred to as a "Back of the Pack'er." We're the ones who feel the nips of the race sweepers at our heels, threatening to wipe us off the course for not finishing in time. We are the *casual* runners, as opposed to the *competitive* runners. *Casual* makes it sound like it's my choice. Like I'm just keeping things casual with running. Like running and I sometimes see other people, because we're non-committal like that.

I didn't run track growing up—in fact, I never even ran a mile without stopping until college. I ran my first 5K in 2002, just because a U.S. President was running it. But somewhere along the way I became addicted. Road races, trail races, obstacle courses—I've tried them all. I've completed runs in every distance category up to a full marathon, and yet I still struggle to call myself "a runner," because I don't look the part, I'm not consistent, and I'm definitely not fast.

I'll admit that I probably like running races because I'm a "Goldfish Poodle." This is a term my friend Amy and I came up with to describe my general state of being. There is a myth that goldfish only have a three-second memory span, and so every lap of their fishbowl is like seeing the world for the first time. I'm typically moving so quickly through life that I feel that way, too. I'm easily excited and love to find fun wherever possible, which also makes me seem like a hyper poodle. The term Goldfish Poodle was born to describe me in the frequent moments when I Have No Idea Where I Am, But I'm Excited About It.

I often feel that way in the middle of races.

So, yes, one reason I keep running might be that my "goldfish" brain forgets how much of a pain the last run was. More than likely it's because my "poodle" brain craves the adventures that happen during training and racing. Days-long relays, obstacle courses involving fire and barbed wire, races at night, races where you wear tutus. (Fact: that can be *every* race, if you want it to be.)

Some adventures can be intimidating, but it's still fun to conquer something new. Plus, if nothing else, after you go through something challenging you end up with great stories. And once you've had one race adventure, you end up wanting that feeling again, so you sign up for more.

The excitement, the fun, and promise of a good story later are a big part of why I keep doing races. But there's more to it. Some part of why I keep running is practical–I have to train if I'm going to run in a race. And, believe me, I need a variety of tricks to keep myself out there. But a bigger part of why I still do it is the rewards I get from running, and from the running community.

Running has helped me deal with coworkers and break-ups, has taught me what I'm capable of physically and emotionally, has introduced me to some fascinating people, and has taught me how to accept support. Of course, it's also gotten me electrocuted....

Chapter 1

HOW IT STARTED

» Swing Set Failures «

"The most effective way to do it is to do it."

AMELIA EARHART

I'm not naturally athletic.

I grew up as more of a book nerd. So much so, that in elementary school I was in what was called the Highly Capable Class. That was the actual name of it, back before our world was full of political correctness. Since we were in grade school, I can only imagine that *highly capable* meant I was marginally less likely to eat glue. In any case, while I was apparently considered highly capable of passing second grade, I was never considered highly capable of becoming a professional athlete.

I remember one afternoon vividly, the one when I was playing on the rings on my swing set, trying to somehow flip over while only using one ring. (Don't ask me why I needed to do this. I grew up in the middle of orchards in eastern Washington, so unless I wanted to play in irrigation systems, my entertainment options were limited.) I managed to flip over enough to get stuck upside down with one leg on either side of the metal chain attaching the ring to the top of the swing set—and said chain was now hitting me like a thong Speedo. I clearly couldn't flip over any further, unless I let the chain split my torso in half vertically, and that seemed too time-consuming. So instead I let go of the ring and fell directly onto the ground below, head first. This example illustrates both my incredible stubbornness in achieving personal goals, and my incredible misunderstanding of physics and kinesthesia.

Years later, I joined a basketball team because a) I'm

tall, and thus the world demands I try to be a basketball player, and b) I was the kid who never sat still and who begged my parents until they agreed to piano lessons, dance lessons, softball, *and* basketball, on top of my candidacy for fifth-grade class president, the pursuit of my creative vision for a class-wide dance routine, and my development of a school newspaper while I recovered from an appendectomy. (My parents obviously deserve a medal.) While on the basketball team, I learned even more about how naturally bad I was at sports.

I distinctly recall one basketball practice where our coach was teaching us about defense. She told us to stand with our arms crossed over our chests, in front of the person we were guarding, whenever they had the ball. Looking back now, I assume that was to teach us how to avoid fouling, but I really don't know because, as you'll see in a minute, I didn't effectively grasp the concept of basketball in general.

I haven't mentioned yet that what I lack in natural athletic ability, I make up for in being extremely literal and inclined to follow orders. So when I was told to stand, that's what I did. Even after the person I was guarding ran toward the basket, I stood, alone, facing my original direction, arms folded across my chest. It didn't take me long to realize that couldn't possibly be the right thing to do. Eventually, I ran after the person I was supposed to be guarding, but the fact that I *know* I stood there being ineffective for those few seconds makes that one of the painful moments confirming that I don't inherently "get" sports.

Instead of playing basketball in high school, I ended up on the dance team. Dancing means you get a set of explicit movements to follow, and you're not required to use logic to release yourself from a folded-arms-chest-stance without being specifically instructed to do so. Hence, dancing and I got along well.

I played no sports in college. After graduating, I moved to Washington, D.C. and started working as a staffer in the White House. I quickly realized that the way all those serious, powerful people running the country let off steam was by acting like children and playing things like adult dodgeball after work. I ended up in two kickball leagues, on a couple of flag football teams, and in various softball leagues, in both the Legislative and the Executive branches of government. I was on teams called things like The Department of Homeland Security Rough Riders and The White House Seals—officially named after the Seal of the Executive Office of the President, but we took along a stuffed seal of the mammal variety as our mascot to games. Nerds. All of us.

On all those teams, the position I played was the same: Filling the Girl Quota. To keep things equal and gender-inclusive, there are rules for most recreational sports leagues that stipulate you must have so many females playing, or you're penalized. Even though I was a member of all those teams, I knew I wasn't being welcomed for my athleticism.

There are no Girl Quotas in running. So while I could justify my existence on a team by the fact that my bathroom symbol wears a skirt, I couldn't do that when I started running races. I had to convince myself that I had a right to be on a course, even if I was never going to break the finish line tape.

D.C. is full of runners, so it's easy to get sucked in, even if you're terrible. During my first year there, President Bush created a 5K race for about 200 people. I decided to do it, because how can you say no to running with Secret Service agents? My FOMO is too strong. (FOMO = Fear of Missing Out. This fear has lead me to all kinds of races, dangerous trips overseas, living on a music tour bus, having a topless Turkish woman bathe me in public, and eventually joining the U.S. military. My FOMO feels a little excessive and should probably be addressed before I really hurt myself.) That 5K was my first race, and I've been hooked ever since.

> **PRO TIP:** Even if you made it into adulthood without running, you aren't out of the woods yet. You may still get sucked in.

I ran another 5K race a year or so later, when I was working for Governor Mitch Daniels, then the director of the White House Office of Management and Budget. I probably had no business being out there in that race, but I can't resist being a part of a team when the opportunity presents itself. Plus, a Management and Budget office doesn't sound like it would be full of jocks. It turned out, however, that the governor was fast, his legislative aide was fast, and even the scrawny staffer on our team who showed up to the race wearing glasses and jeans was fast. And then there was me, who was eventually passed by a senator who was 107 years old if he was a day.

I was also passed by a pregnant lady and a man wearing goggles. I quickly learned to embrace the fact that I will be passed. A lot. So I might as well be amused by it.

> **PRO TIP:** Being slow allows you to enjoy the parade of people who pass you. Sometimes it's a hot man, sometimes it's an octogenarian. Either way, it's a nice distraction from sweating.

I did one more 5K before jumping full-on into The Army Ten-Miler. The ATM is a favorite in D.C., and while I'll run three miles for Secret Service agents, apparently I'll run ten for soldiers. Another trend in my running career (that I'm just now realizing) is the lure of the inclusion of attractive men. I ran the Nike Women's Half Marathon last year with a four-pound tumor in my abdomen because they promised a fireman would be handing out the race medals at the end. If nothing else, I'm rewards-driven.

You might wonder how I decided I could even run ten miles without ever having done it before. I'll tell you how: I'd heard friends say they'd run that race, and I remember immediately sizing them up and secretly thinking, *She looks like she's fond of simple carbohydrates and reality television marathons too. If she can do it, I should be able to.*

> **PRO TIP:** Find someone similar to you—in size, ability, addiction to cheese, etc.—who has run a race. If they can do it, you can, too.

I don't remember much about that first ten-miler, except that I didn't train well, I finished, and I was sore afterwards. But it was a good sore. An empowering sore. I know what you're thinking: *Sure, "empowering," like how women say drugless births are "empowering."* But don't worry. I almost never feel like I'm giving birth while running a race.

Side note: Can we just talk about why birth has been deemed the thing to do without drugs? No one says, "Get a root canal without Novocain—it's empowering," yet women have latched on (no breastfeeding pun intended) to this idea of natural births and now we all have to keep up, amiright ladies? Or it might just be me who feels like I now need to keep up. But then again, if she can do it...

Side note to the side note: Speaking of natural births, my friend used her race experience to prepare for her birth: "I worked for 7 hours in my half Ironman, so I know I can do labor up to that point. After that, who knows..." So I suppose that's another motivation to do a race, if you need one: It will help you prepare for that no-Novocain child delivery you're going to end up doing because everyone else is. (Before the proponents of natural child birth attack me, I do realize that there are health benefits and good reasons, etc., etc., but I also think some people do natural child birth as a trend and that puts a lot of pressure on me, because I'm someone who likes to be trendy.)

Somewhere around 2004, I misplaced my sense of self-preservation and decided to attempt a half marathon. I signed up for The Rock 'n' Roll Half Marathon in Virginia Beach, Virginia. (I was probably subconsciously lured in by the thought of male lifeguards.) I was spectacularly underprepared, as was my race partner Rebekah, and, honestly, we didn't even think we would finish. When the race started, we kept ourselves distracted for a good few miles by joking about how far we thought we could actually go, and then making up ridiculous "ratios" that made no sense but kept us entertained. "We could start with a 1/1..." (meaning run one *mile*, walk one *minute*) "... for the first 5K..." (three-ish miles) "... and a 2/1..." (meaning run two *minutes*, walk one minute) "... for one mile, and a 1/2 for the next two miles...." We actually made it to mile seven without taking any walk breaks, because we were so busy trying to do math while pretending there was a chance we'd actually finish at all.

At mile seven, the sun hit me like kryptonite and I melted to a walk, while Rebekah continued on. I caught up to her later and we finished the race by alternating between walking and running each mile to the finish. Around mile 11, I got overzealous with hydration. Around mile 13, I got overzealous with "finishing strong" and started hurrying toward the end.

If you've ever tried chugging liquid and then sprinting, you probably see where this is going. As I crossed the finish line (the finish was videotaped), I turned to my left to slap hands with Rebekah in victory...

... then turned to my right to vomit.

So, if you enjoy uncontrollably losing the contents of your stomach in front of strangers, racing without training might be for you. I'm afraid this experience became sort of a standing challenge for me through my twenties, like, "If I can do *that* without training, imagine what other kinds of puke-inducing activities I might be able to barely make it through!"

Really, though, it was pure laziness that prevented me from consistently training. Once I knew I could finish a race without much preparation, that's what I did. I'd be slow during a race and I'd be sore afterwards, but the races themselves were still fun.

PRO TIP: Get a friend to join you in a race, one who prepares just as poorly and runs just as slowly as you. Then it's like you're simply hanging out together, except you both smell and you're both in pain.

Races are grand events, often with music and cheering fans and a ton of people around slogging along too. You find your part of the pack and feel included in something. I may not instinctually understand sports, but I can put one foot in front of the other and follow a race course (if it's well-marked, and roped off, and has some sort of alert system in case I start to veer off in the wrong direction).

As a little, bookish kid, I didn't always think like the other kids around me and I didn't always play like they did. But when I grew up and started running in races, I realized I could belong. I was doing what everyone else was doing. I had a race bib too, which meant I was part of the club. It didn't matter if I under-prepared—I still wanted to race, because of what it gave me.

PRO TIP: Running will welcome you, no matter how highly incapable you've been at sports. Give it the chance to do that.

Eventually—after something broke in my head in 2010 and I decided to run a full marathon—I did learn how much better it is when I consistently train.

According to runningusa.org, there has been a 40 percent increase in U.S. marathon finishers over the past decade. Maybe that's because so many of us have desk jobs and either need to exercise or need to prove to the world that we can do more than create pivot tables in an Excel spreadsheet (which I can't actually do, so I now have two things I need to prove to the world). I spent years saying I'd never run a full marathon and righteously informing people that "the human body is not meant to run 26 miles." (Listen to the girl who doesn't understand how swing sets work—she probably knows what she's talking about.)

Then I was a bridesmaid, and my feelings about the level of stress I was willing to put on my body changed when I realized I wanted to lose weight. The bride was Tiffani, who was one of my best friends from college. We had spent a semester in Europe together where we made it through lost luggage in Italy, trains detaching unexpectedly in France, and the unfortunate necessity of using a private field as a bathroom while squatting near a bull in the middle of Ireland (okay, that incident might have only happened to me, but Tiffani was an accomplice). Situations like that have made me less fearful of embarrassment, which has been helpful in some of my running experiences. Naturally, Tiffani and I were bonded enough for me to want to be in her wedding.

As Tiffani's big day approached, I clearly remember talking

to the other bridesmaids about how small the dresses ran. "I mean I had to get mine *two whole sizes* bigger than my normal size!" I said. Those silly dressmakers were obviously at fault.

It wasn't until later that I realized I actually *was* two sizes bigger than I'd thought, and had been stretching my clothes and living in denial. As I looked critically at the wedding photos later, I resolved to lose weight, even if it killed me (or broke up my long-term relationship with caramel mochas, which was equally undesirable).

I decided to order Nutrisystem weight-loss products, because Marie Osmond is made of happiness and promise, and she's very hard to say no to. But then I felt like I needed to add a fitness goal to my Magical Osmond Meal Plan, so I researched marathon training teams. With that, my once-casual relationship with running was about to transition to "it's complicated."

....

MORAL OF THE STORY:

Running is welcoming to even the least athletically inclined, but it's also a sneaky little drug that will— like caramel mochas—keep you coming back for more. Lace up and enjoy the ride.

Chapter 2

THE MARATHON
» Wardrobe Malfunctions and «
Pacing Senior Citizens

"No doubt a brain and some shoes are essential for marathon success, although if it comes down to a choice, pick the shoes. More people finish marathons with no brains than with no shoes."

DON KARDONG

I honestly don't remember how I decided on a marathon as my weight-loss enabler. I searched through old emails and found one I'd written on November 15, 2009, to my friend Kami. The subject line just said, "Marathon," and the email started with, "I may want to do one. Haha."

I bet that's exactly how Neil Armstrong informed his friends about his decision to go into space. "Moon landing. I may want to do one. Haha."

My email went on to ask Kami if she was interested in doing it with me. Since she and I have done everything together, from dodging swine flu in Nicaragua to smearing natural hot spring mud on our faces and dancing in a water party in Iceland, I figured she'd be an easy target.

She wasn't. She didn't even reply to my email.

The next day, I tried to convince Rebekah—the friend I'd nearly puked on in the half marathon—and she declined. My pitch to her had been: "I'm considering training for a marathon next year!! Any interest? I know I said I never wanted to, but a friend was talking me into it and she said it really only hurts your Friday night social life and I hardly ever do much on Fridays anyway!"

My reasoning behind wanting to do this marathon thing was ironclad.

The day after that, I sent an email to another friend, ending with, "I'm considering running a marathon in Nashville on April 24th... LOL." (I was always dying laughing talking about this marathon idea. That should've been a sign that I had lost my senses and should not have been allowed to sign up for anything.)

Two days later, I emailed myself:

From: *Dana Ayers*

To: *Dana Ayers*

Date: *Thu, Nov 19, 2009 at 9:10 AM*

Subject: *Q's for Marathon*

How many miles do I need to run during the week (prob have to do treadmill)?

How much do I have to pay/raise?

What's schedule—really cold? How long for run/ walk in race, etc.

My thought process is just begging for dissection. First off, the question that's totally missing: "*Will I die?*" Second, what's with the treadmill aside to myself? Did I believe Americans were only allowed so many miles on the road and the rest were mandated for inside? Did I think I'd later forget that treadmills existed, and so felt I should remind my future self that they would be an option?

The next issue that concerned me was money. That

must have been after I'd looked into charity fundraising training teams and become more concerned about the cost of purchasing my suffering than the fact that I was *volunteering* to purchase suffering.

Finally, I expressed interest in the training schedule (which should've been near the top of my list) and concern about whether it was going to be really cold. I don't know who I thought I could ask that question to—Our Maker, perhaps? In which case, again, there were so many more questions I should've lined up first, like "Why did You design me with an interest in paying for self-torture?" and "What was Your purpose in creating people who think toilet paper should be pulled from underneath the roll?"

With those and other questions lingering in my mind, on Dec 1, 2009, I attended an information session for Team in Training (TNT), the national race-training program that raises money for leukemia and lymphoma research. I went to the session alone, but immediately ran into Lauren, someone I'd worked with years earlier and hadn't seen since. I had no clue she ran at all, and definitely didn't know she coached for TNT. (Lauren once sent an email asking me to call a repairman for the office copier because "The error message says it has 'mechanical problems.' As opposed to 'emotional' or 'spiritual' problems." I liked her after that email.) I took seeing her at this event as a good sign.

After listening to the information presented in the session, I had the type of moment I've had a few times since.

It's that moment when you're about to make a decision that's so crazy you step outside yourself and watch yourself do it in slow motion. That moment of deciding to "*Push the button!*" All you can do afterward is strap in and enjoy whatever ride on which you're about to be taken. In that moment at the TNT information session, I signed a commitment to raise (or pay) $3,000 in return for receiving marathon training for the Rock 'n' Roll Country Music Marathon in Nashville.

What did I just do?

> **PRO TIP:** "Adulting" can be boring. Sometimes we need to shock our systems by jumping in and committing to something, and worrying about the how part later.

For the next five months, I woke up early every Saturday to run anywhere from four to 20 miles with my training team—in rain, shine, or snow (yes, Past Self, it *was* going to be "really cold"). I trained during the year of the D.C. "Snowpocalypse," where we got record-breaking snow-falls that shut down the federal government. I remember running when our water bottles froze, and when I told myself the icy winds hitting me in the face were giving me some sort of power burst. I became delusional.

Running for a cause helped, though. We had team meetings, we got emails that told us about the lives improved through TNT's funds for cancer research, and we even had one Team member who ran with us during the course of his own cancer treatment. It's hard to complain about icy wind after that.

I consistently followed the program for the entire five months, often waking up before work to get my training in. We were given a schedule to follow, and tips on nutrition, hydration, and stretching along the way. Our training was to do a combination of different things: about three days a week of "short" runs (ranging from two to five miles, and varying in intensity—sometimes we were to run hills, sometimes we were to run faster than our normal pace, etc.), a "long" run once a week (this was the only training done as a group; the rest of the training we did on our own), cross-training days (something besides running, to keep up fitness and to stretch and strengthen different muscles), and rest days (I was the best at these).

I can barely believe I did it, to be honest. Right now, the thought of waking up early to run before work sounds like something I could never maintain. But I *did,* so now I have no excuse to ever say I *can't.* This is one of the risks of training and racing–you may injure the excuses part of your brain. Mine's irreparable. For example, I now know I can keep my body in motion for five and a half hours, because that's the time it took for me to finish my marathon (slower than Oprah, but right around Katie Holmes. And that's a pretty good position in life in general, I think.) I also know I can find the will to get up early and work out on a consistent basis. I can't tell myself *I can't* anymore. It's a terrible injury, really. Super annoying.

I accidentally learned a lot through those five months of training. I started gaining interest in things like "carb-loading" and "the importance of a strong core." I found myself Googling "injury prevention" and "foam rollers" in my spare time. I didn't intend to become a fitness and nutrition guru, but that was one surprising side effect of Operation I Just Need Something to Force Me to Move My Body before Pool Covers and REI Tents are My Only Clothing Options.

One of the things I learned was that training is not always about the running itself, but about getting "time on your feet," meaning that it's beneficial to simply keep your body in motion for the length of time it will take you to run a race. I learned that you never need to train up to the full length of a race, because adrenaline will carry you through the last two to six miles. I also learned that chafing can occur under butt cheeks, and that you won't learn it happened until you shower later. And then you will cry.

I learned that sunscreen also acts as a great skin protector in freezing winds, and that body temperature rises 20 degrees when you get going, so you need to wear less clothing than you'd think. I also learned about Gina's dating life, Becky's mom who passed away from cancer, and Ashley's history as a weight-lifter. When I started,

I didn't know anyone in the group except Lauren, but when you hit the trail for hours with people, you get to know them really well.

Throughout that whole season, I kept worrying that I'd get injured and be unable to finish the race. Thankfully, I made it through almost the entire training program without a big mishap. Then we did our longest training run—a 20-miler—and that's when it happened, my almost injury.

I was running with Gina, and we got to around mile 13 and she wanted to stop at a convenience store we were passing. I hardly ever stopped on training runs. I'm slow enough as it is. I don't need to waste time. But since she stopped, I stopped. And since we were there, I went ahead and used the restroom, not knowing what that indulgence was about to cost me. The yoga pants I was wearing were many years old and well-worn. So as I pulled them up... they ripped.

Not just a little rip, but like a good 6–8 inch tear down the seam.

And not just any seam.

I tore the seam running along the inside of my thigh, starting a bit above my knee and going almost all the way up to Victoria's Secret.

I was dumbfounded. We were miles from our cars and I had no cell phone or wallet on me. I walked out of the

bathroom, pointed out the incident in disbelief to Gina—
as if she couldn't already see it—and asked the cashier if
he had anything that could help me. Safety pins? Tape?
I would've stapled the material to my flesh at that point
to get back to my car. But he had nothing useful for me,
and the line of people waiting to purchase items started
building, so he ignored us. Gina and I began to forage the
aisles for tape.

But we had no money.

So here's where I sort of stole something. I'm not proud
of what I did, but panic set in. It was either murder Gina
and take her pants, or find a roll of masking tape, duck
behind an aisle, peel off enough to wrap around my leg,
tourniquet-style, toss the tape back on the shelf, and
scurry out of the store. Those were obviously the only
two options I had.

We got back on the trail and my MacGyver-ed pant leg
was still sort of gaping, but *whatever*, it was working. Sort
of. Except every couple minutes, the tape shifted and the
hole started to open again. So I had to keep readjusting,
and the tape steadily rubbed a large area raw on the inside
of my thigh.

Around mile 18, we had the choice of running straight
to our cars or going another two miles to finish the 20
miles we were supposed to do. Gina decided to turn
toward the cars, but I was all, "*No. Way*. I've just run
the last five miles looking like a bad war movie extra,

stopping every couple minutes to yank a hole closed on my pants. *I am finishing this!*"

I ran the last bit dealing with weird looks from other runners, and finally rounded the bend and got back to where my car was. The stragglers who were left of my training team started cheering for me. Then they saw my leg and I had to explain myself. One teammate mused, "Oh, I saw the tape but figured it was some sort of circulation-improvement thing or something." That's how crazy runners are.

> **PRO TIP:** Even in the midst of struggle (and perhaps humiliation), something primal inside rises up to finish a run. Harness that drive and you can use it later when you have to do other uncomfortable things in life, like finish your taxes (which we can all agree is overwhelming, whether your pants remain intact or not).

When I got home from that training run, my leg was chafed so badly I was unable to run the next week, which made that my worst "injury" all season.

But that wasn't where the adventures ended.

A couple weeks later, we finally finished our training and arrived in Nashville for the race. The excitement was off the charts. TNT does it right, and they had a welcome dinner where we walked past dozens of people cheering for us on our way to a nice meal and a last-minute pep talk.

On the day of the race, our training team was wearing our pre-planned race-day outfits. We'd eaten and slept properly. We were ready to do this.

Then a tornado arrived.

Literally, a freak storm rolled towards Nashville. The weather channel reported a tornado warning for the area where the marathon was being held. We started the race anyway, running past fans holding ominous signs, like "Run faster than the storm!" We kept praying we could.

At the halfway point of the marathon, we were diverted off the planned route and had to finish there.

After all those months of training, that news was heart-breaking. Some people kept running laps in the parking lot until they finished 26 miles on their own, others just teared up in disappointment (ok that may have just been me, until my running partner and former-soldier friend basically told me to suck it up and shamed me out of it. Girls can be so nurturing.)

We got through a very anti-climactic finish, flew back home, and some of us frantically searched for other marathon options near us that we could finish before we lost the value of our hard work of training.

To further complicate things, I had pre-planned a trip

to Turkey and Greece for immediately after Nashville, to celebrate a friend's birthday. I barely had time to shoot off an email begging the Delaware Marathon for late entry before I flew overseas.

My trip to Greece occurred during deadly riots in Athens, so the day I got word via the computer in our hotel lobby that Delaware was going to let me run, I had just returned from dodging bombed-out buildings, vehicle fires, and tear-gas. This marathon thing was getting more exciting by the minute!

I finally returned home. My vacation had included no running at all the previous week, during which time I'd embraced a diet of copious amounts of baklava and spanakopita. It probably wouldn't be pretty, but I was still going to do this marathon. A week after my return to the U.S., I headed to Delaware.

I had now gone from being in a famous race of 30,000 runners in Nashville to being in the 7th annual 649-runner marathon in Wilmington, Delaware. If I didn't get it right this time, odds were I'd be finishing my first marathon by running alone back and forth between the Capitol Building and the Lincoln Memorial until the park police became suspicious. *This better work.*

Two other TNT girls who couldn't finish Nashville and I went to Wilmington together. The race offered an early start for slower runners, and I chose that so my teammates wouldn't have to wait so long for me to finish. *Ah, pace.*

You keep me so humble.

After leaving our hotel later than planned, I was dropped off on a corner, practically tucked and rolled out of the car, and then scampered over to the start line. There were 30 to 40 other early starters—mostly senior citizens. I had a few minutes to swallow my pride and start making friends before we took off.

"Taking off" probably isn't the most appropriate term, considering we could have sipped tea at the pace we were going. But being slow has its perks. Races are like mullets: business in the front, party in the back. Back there, everyone chats. I met a nice 62-year-old man named Roscoe, from Macon, Georgia, who told me about his four kids and that he was doing *two marathons a month* that year until he finished marathons in all 50 states. There were actually several runners who had already done marathons in all 50 states—sometimes three times over. Most were over 60.

> **PRO TIP:** If you worry you can't finish a marathon, remember that there are grandparents out there right now running their second one this month (and I'm probably running at their pace). This means you can run one too.

I stayed with Roscoe while we tried to figure out the

course. There were three races going on simultaneously in Wilmington: our marathon, a relay race, and a half-marathon. If that wasn't enough to confuse me, the marathon course basically consisted of running the half-marathon course twice. I assume this was because Wilmington is so small they couldn't find 26 consecutive miles for us.

Parts of the course went through desolate areas with few markings. Two different times, Roscoe and I thought we'd missed a turn. And because of the two loops and three races, we were constantly running by signs like "Mile 3!" (for the marathoners), followed by a sign that said "Relay turnaround!" followed by a sign that said "Mile 16!" (for those in the second lap of the marathon). It's a miracle I didn't get lost or take off in the wrong direction.

We started running around 6:20 a.m. I had chosen to do the Jeff Galloway "Run Walk" method for the race, which meant I would run for so many minutes, then take a one minute walk break, then repeat. This was before iPhones or popular fitness watches, so I used a Gymboss timer ("Gymmy" for short) to time my ratios. Gymmy clipped to my belt and would beep at me when it was time to start walking or running again. We were very close.

The regular start for the marathon was 7 a.m. By 7:40, I was already getting passed by runners who started after me. Shortly after that, I was passed by a man wearing a tutu. A new low. Shortly after that: Gymmy stopped working. *Traitor*.

Fortunately, I had also borrowed my coach's watch, so I spent the rest of the race constantly checking to make sure I stayed on my run/walk ratio. Once again, I used my terrible math skills as a distraction while I tried to keep up with how long I'd been running overall.

At mile 15, I passed Roscoe again after I had stopped to use a Porta-Potty.

Throughout the race, I was also getting lapped by regular marathoners, the faster relay runners, and even race leaders who had motorcycle escorts. So not only was I doing math in my head, trying to stay on the right course, and singing "Yellow Submarine" to myself because I didn't have an iPod (and because I tend to fixate on weird songs when I run long distances), I also had to sidestep a motorcycle-escorted fast runner every few miles. Humbling.

I was encouraged, however, by the nice locals cheering us on. A few times during the course, Lauren or another TNT coach would find me and run for a while and other TNT members from all over the country would yell my name (printed on my tank top) and encourage me as well. At times near the end, I was tempted to stop running, but I never stopped smiling.

Mile 26 came out of nowhere and as I ran across the finish, I started to feel like I would burst into tears.

Then I felt like I might throw up.

Not again ....

Fortunately, neither happened. I finished triumphantly, and the race photographers got some awesome shots of me and my bulging thigh muscles. So I *did* lose weight during this marathon-running process, but since I also gained muscle it didn't quite work as well as I hoped for getting thin. I did look more intimidating to my desk job coworkers, though, so some good came out of it. I've also now been on an extremely awkward date where I managed to sit with a new guy on my left, while my ex was two seats to my right. (Don't ask. These things just happen to me—like tornados and riots.) The new guy commented, "You have nice quads." So while that's not the most romantic thing to hear on a date, and my ex probably had a great laugh at my expense, it is affirming to know that running gives you more than just blisters.

Looking back on that whole challenging process, I only have happy feelings. So often in life, things mean more after they happen than while they occur. That's when you realize it's what the thing represents that made the biggest impact. That race in Wilmington, and all the long months of training beforehand, represents my ability to be strong, to not whine, to finish what I start, and to make a personal dream a reality.

> **PRO TIP:** Running offers the opportunity to prove ourselves. We aren't just going to an event to observe, we're making our bodies obey us and accomplish something.

That time of marathon training also represents the friendships I formed with others who were choosing to get out and do something, to challenge their own excuses—people like Gina, who convinced me two years later to do another race I said I'd never do—Tough Mudder. That one involved obstacles. It would also involve another tornado, as you're about to find out.

....

MORAL OF THE STORY:

It really is possible to achieve a big goal like finishing a marathon, even without being super fit, super fast, or super athletic. We are capable of way more than we think we are—we just need to find the spaces in which to prove ourselves. Like on the road, running next to a grandpa from Georgia named Roscoe.

Chapter 3

THE TOUGH MUDDER

» Paying To Sign a Death Waiver «

"I am always doing things I can't do—that's how I get to do them."

PABLO PICASSO

Before I did it, I said the same thing about Tough Mudder that I'd said about running a marathon: "I'll never do one."

Tough Mudder is a "challenge" involving running around for miles and completing about 26 obstacles along the way. I had run a few obstacle course races before, but most were only about three miles long. Tough Mudder was about 12 miles long, and was touted as something only the fiercest people could finish. The ads for it talked about the dozens of "hard core" obstacles "created by British Special Forces." I briefly checked in with my soul to see if we were hard core enough to try it, and the answer was a resounding "Nope!" I regarded Tough Mudder as something only *really* fit people do, not something that I, and my mostly casual relationship with running, should attempt.

Then, in 2012, Gina—who had helped me tape my pants back together during marathon training—told me she was training for her second Tough Mudder and I should join her team. Once again, I was lured in by my belief that if a friend had completed something without dying, I could probably do it too. (This belief doesn't include friends who become Navy SEALs, free-climb rock faces, or give up gluten. I don't care if they succeed, those things would totally kill me.) I also realized there's a cumulative effect from having multiple successes. Each race I finished layered on top of the other ones in my memory bank to form a combined little mound of confidence that said, "There's a small chance you could survive Tough Mudder without perishing or mangling yourself entirely." That was good enough for me.

> **PRO TIP:** Race successes build on top of each other and bolster your confidence. If you're not careful, you begin consistently doing things you said you'd never do.

I joined Gina's Tough Mudder training team, which was made up of people she knew from her gym, and included a couple of personal trainers and a few former Marines. I felt like they might either whip me into shape or wash me out in some kind of hazing event if they felt I couldn't hack it. Either way, I trusted their judgment.

The training consisted of working out on our own through the week, then coming together as a group on Sundays to run around Great Falls National Park on the banks of the Potomac River in Virginia. There, our team captain would have us simulate various things we might face in Mudder while confused hikers looked on. We practiced low-crawling through the grass, we chased each other over downed trees, and we hoisted ourselves up and over the walls of the dried-up boat locks of the Patowmack Canal. We got our feet wet in the Potomac to practice running in soggy socks. You know, normal stuff.

PRO TIP: If nothing else, training and racing can arm you with interesting material for social media posts or when answering the age-old question, "So, what did you do this weekend?"

I loved being part of a team and training with my Tough Mudder teammates, and I liked pushing myself. It felt good to be outside and working new muscles. I was surprised to find that I could actually keep up with the group, for the most part. As we got closer to the event, I felt fairly prepared.

Then I made the mistake of researching reviews of the event and looking through past participants' photos of the obstacles. I saw images of grown men wearing expressions of teething-infant-level howling as they were hit by electricity from the mass of hanging wires they ran through. I saw people preparing to jump off a ledge, appearing to be near bladder failure with fear. The reviews said things like, "The worst that those electric wires will do is shut down your body and make you poop yourself. Otherwise, you're all good." We had *not* practiced that. Perhaps this was a bad idea after all.

My team and I arrived on race day not sure what to expect. The forecast for the day was for temperatures in the 80s, with 85 percent humidity and a chance of thunderstorms. The race location was on farmland that took entirely too long to get to in all the event traffic, making us miss our actual start time, forcing us to start later than we'd planned. On top of all this, the event coordinators made us sign *death waivers,* and they wrote our bib numbers on our foreheads so "We can identify your body later, if need be."

My team headed to the start line to receive final words (that term means more when you've literally just signed a death waiver) from the race emcee. We proceeded to get the best pep talk I've ever had before a race. It included compliments about our braveness and getting us to yell several rounds of "*Hoo*-rah!" at various statements. At one point, we chanted and waved our hands collectively, hip-hop-hooray style, and I smiled and wondered, *Did I just accidentally join a cult?* We were told to "take a knee" and the motivational speech continued, except now intermixed with buzz-kill warnings from our emcee:

"Now be careful out there—we've already had people hurt."

"We've already seen sprained ankles, dislocated knees."

"Someone's already bit through their lip from the electric shocks."

"If you can't swim—*skip the water obstacles.* You all laugh, but there'll be someone who does it anyway—and you will need to pull that person out."

"Enjoy this time now, 'cause pain's coming!"

I felt like I had enough motivation, and silently willed the emcee to let us start before I changed my mind. With a plume of Tough Mudder orange ceremonial smoke rushing at us, that's finally what we did.

Our first obstacle was called Arctic Enema, so you can imagine the level of enjoyment it brought. I found myself jumping into an icy pool, gasping uncontrollably, and pawing the now water-splotched and ineffective sunglasses off my face. It wasn't enough to immerse our organs in icy water, we had to completely submerge and swim *under* something (don't ask me what that something was, because I was fairly blacked-out by that point) and come up, half-panicked from the inability to inhale, on the other side of the obstacle, then continue swimming until we could pull ourselves out. Everyone's faces resembled that famous Edvard Munch painting *The Scream,* but at least our adrenaline was pumping already.

We proceeded through various other obstacles, including one that was a series of ditches we were supposed to jump over. Sounds easy, right? Except the ground was mud. And the ditches were filled with more mud. So, no matter what we did, we were pretty much going to slip in mud.

Some of the people on our team leapt over the mud ditch, slid to the ground on top of the rise when they landed, but then jumped back up to try to "catch" the next person leaping. I panicked and pictured the pulled muscles I was going to get right off the bat by landing in a tangle of my own splayed-out giraffe limbs. I didn't give it enough gas when I took flight and ended up planting myself against the bank I was supposed to land on top of, legs half in the ditch of mud, arms pulled on by my laughing teammates, while they asked if I was ok. Even with that lack of grace, I still fared better than our team captain, whose right leg made it onto the top of the bank—but his left leg didn't. That landing position left him basically castrated on the side of the bank before he slid woefully into the muddy ditch, while people commented that they hoped he'd already had kids.

We finally all made it out of the ditches, covered in mud, with several miles left to run. To make things even more interesting, I had the worst head cold I'd had in years and, let me tell you, besides not being able to breathe normally, it's not easy going through a race where everything is muddy and you need to blow your nose. I used a *banana peel* as a tissue at one of the refreshment stops. That was a new low. At one point, I looked at a teammate and asked, "Is there mud and snot dried on my face right now?" I got a matter-of-fact, "Yes." And on we ran.

We carried logs for a quarter mile. We entered caves before knowing what was in them. We swam through muddy water and low-crawled under barbed wire—which basically looks like slithering through mud like lizards. This race is where vanity goes to die.

We arrived at one obstacle that required us to shimmy into what resembled long, human-sized bendy straws. I inched myself through one, my face following some stranger's rear end ahead of me, and my mind filling with questions like, "Am I claustrophobic? Why didn't I ask myself this before I got here?" One of my former-Marine teammates managed to get wedged into his straw until he could no longer proceed on his own and had to be pulled out by his girlfriend. We would all lose little pieces of our pride before the day was done.

> **PRO TIP:** Don't be afraid to flounder. Even tough Marine dudes struggle in endurance challenges and have to be rescued by their significant others.

Eventually our team made it through the straws and ran towards the next obstacle, called Electric Eel. I saw where this was going. We had to low-crawl—*through water*—under electric wires. *Seriously, does the government know this race is allowed to happen?* The shocks from accidentally touching the wires seemed to hit people at random. Thankfully, none of us felt much more than a faint buzzing, except for the team member who had metal staples in her body–no shock there! (I will not apologize for that pun.) I decided the purpose of the Electric Eel was to add another level of psychological stress.

You know what else will do that? When they close an obstacle because they're looking for a body. Which is what we were told at another obstacle as we watched paramedics and guys in scuba gear head into the water. I'm pretty sure the person in trouble ended up safe, but we didn't know that until later. So that added to our duress, as did the official signage along the course stating things like, "Remember, you signed a death waiver," and "If you're tired now, you're in trouble." In fact, I don't remember exactly what that sign said, because I *was* already tired by that point.

They ended up having to close other water obstacles later because of a massive thunderstorm that rolled in—as if the course wasn't difficult enough, Mother Nature got involved. Apparently, electrocuting us was ok if the Tough Mudder people did it, but was deemed "unsafe" if we were electrocuted by natural causes. When those obstacles closed, a crazy thing happened. Everyone started protesting to the race staff, saying things like, "*But we signed a death waiver!*" That's what happens to your brain when you get into a racing adventure. The thrill of it all takes over your survival instinct.

There were plenty of other obstacles to keep us busy, however, even without the ones that closed. There were giant walls to scale, enormous stacks of hay bales to climb. And then, the highest obstacle of all: Walk the Plank. The plank was a high ledge we were to jump off of into water below. I tried to find a stat on the height of the plank, but all the event website said was "15+ feet."

15 plus *what*? 10 more feet? Death?

All I know is it was *high*. So high that some people

had second thoughts. I made the lifeguard promise she wouldn't let anyone land on top of me after I jumped, and as soon as I felt sure there were no poor souls in the water directly below me, I stepped off.

And immediately realized what a long pause it was.

Just me. Hanging out in the air. Falling... still... falling....

"What did I just do?"

That's the thought I distinctly remember having right before I finally let out a strangled scream halfway down. In retrospect, it's the thought we all *should've* had right after agreeing to do this race in the first place, had we any sense. But, *eh*. You live and learn. Or, you hope you live anyway.

We all survived the Plank and went on through some more obstacles until we came upon one that turned out to be a favorite of mine. For the most part. Until it went on forever and got old, which most of the obstacles did. (I'm *still* crawling? I'm *still* jumping over ditches? I'm *still* falling off that stupid plank?)

Let me try to explain this one. I think they called it the Mud Mile. It was a series of giant mounds of mud, with more mud in between (those Tough Mudder people really like to hammer a point home). Unlike the ditch-jumping obstacle, we couldn't leap from mound to mound, because they were too far apart. We had to run straight up them, then slide down the other side, swim through mud, then head up the next mound. And we typically couldn't even run up them, because they were so slippery. We were left to the mercy of strangers to pull us up to the top, before sliding like seals down the other side.

Relying on strangers was one of the best parts about this race, though. We all helped each other. I absolutely planted both hands on both butt cheeks of a perfect stranger during the Mud Mile to push her up one of those mounds. People slid down in all different ways, sometimes face first. I started seeing body parts poking out of the mud at odd angles because of the way people became submerged between the mounds. I'd slither past a couple of legs sticking out here, an arm and a head reaching out of the mud there, then I'd scramble up the next mound.

> **PRO TIP:** If nothing else, races bring people together. Even if it is through a shared sense of helplessness and loss of dignity.

In case it hasn't become obvious yet—this race defeats any aspirations participants may have of looking cute. Besides what my clothes and skin looked like by that point, I could no longer really control how I moved. I remember hearing the big, strapping guy who was next to me during one of the low crawls grunting loudly with each new heave he gave to push himself forward (and he kept it up even after I started giggling at him). Meanwhile, I'd given up the slither move on that low-crawl obstacle and turned on my side, arm out ahead of me, head on my arm, feet shoving myself along like some deranged dog on the carpet. We did whatever it took to get through.

My team completed every obstacle that wasn't shut down by the storm and finally came to Everest, the one I was dreading the most. Everest was a 15-foot-high metal slope that curved upward and inward from the ground to the top. It's basically one side of those half-pipe ramps used in extreme skateboarding and snowboarding events, except it was covered in greasy mud. And we were supposed to run up it, which seemed unnecessarily cruel. The best bet was to run, leap, and hope some stranger already on the top grabbed your arms and pulled you to safety. But this was after we'd all run about 10 miles, survived about 23 other obstacles, and were covered in mud, so the odds of the mechanics of all this not failing were really low.

Then it started to pour rain.

My resolve began to wash away. The ramp had emblazoned across it the words "No Quit in Here," and I thought, *Well, there's quit in* here *if you need some*, as I examined my own constitution. But I got in line and was prepared to give it a shot anyway, because I had made it so far and didn't want to give up yet.

And that's when I found a man's tooth for him, right after he knocked it out.

I was standing in line and saw a guy bleeding on the ramp, asking everyone to help him. So I went over and actually found the tooth he'd just knocked out while attempting his ascent of Everest. The paramedics took him off and I returned to my team, breezing past them, announcing, "I just found a guy's tooth–I'm out!" And that's how I skipped Everest.

My team had an anticlimactic end of the event when the thunderstorm forced everyone to finish as fast as possible, and because the final obstacle was one that had been shut down by the storm. That one was supposed to be a muddy run through more electric wires, but we were told the electricity had been turned off and to simply walk through it to get to the finish line. I made a joke halfway along about how funny it would be if they switched the electricity back on right then, since we were caressing and pushing through the wires like they were a beaded curtain from the 70s, rather than trying to dodge them in fear for our lives. This photo was captured right at that moment:

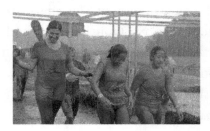

Even though I feel cheated out of some of my experience in the Tough Mudder, and even though the mud was trying to pull my shirt into a kaftan that was clinging to me inappropriately, I do kind of love that photo. (I am the one on the left with the giraffe limbs).

In the end, we all lived. It took us four hours to finish. We crossed the finish line and bought hot dogs that we cradled to protect from the rain until we got to our cars. Then I forgot about mine, stepped on it, found it on the floorboard miles down the road, and ate it anyway. Because that day had turned me into a dude.

We bought dry clothes at the concessions tent, and then later realized the futility of it given that we had to change into our new clothes in the parking lot... in the rain. We made a corporate decision to abandon our sneakers by our cars, as other people had done, because those puppies were never going to come clean.

Then we discovered that we weren't done with obstacles yet. First, we had the challenge of changing clothes. Since we had mud in places where mud *should never be*, we had to strip completely naked to throw on our "dry" (now rainsoaked) outfits. The girls formed dressing huddles and got way more acquainted than we wanted to, then jumped into the cars, only to realize that the parking lot had become, well, a parking lot. Cars were just sitting there, because so many of them were now stuck.

In mud.

Oh, the irony.

We finally got our car out of the lot. As we headed down

the highway, we heard a weather alert saying that not only were we experiencing a crazy storm, but a tornado had been spotted near where we lived. *I should so get extra points for continually having tornados accompany my races.*

I got home to no electricity and prepared to sit on my couch forever, but discovered that was hard to do when no comfortable position existed for my body. I tried to rest my elbows on the table, but they were both scratched. I propped my feet up, but that rubbed the cut on the back of my ankle where pebbles had gotten stuck in my sock and stayed there for the whole race. I tried to cross my legs, but I had bruises on the sides and backs of them and scratches down the fronts. Every now and then, I accidentally grazed the bruise on my hip and fondly remembered torso-planting on the side of that muddy bank.

It was so worth it. I finished something I thought I wasn't tough enough to do. I had such a packed adventure with new friends. I got to wear that silly orange Finisher head-band Tough Mudder gives out, and I got to see people look at me wearing it, probably thinking, *Wow, I've seen those Tough Mudder ads. She must be really hard-core.*

PRO TIP: I'm not really hard-core. I'm afraid of lots of things and I still finished, so don't let race hype intimidate you.

Finishing Tough Mudder made the confidence mound in my head grow even bigger, which meant I'd likely look for another endurance test to attempt. But not anytime soon. First, I wanted to watch TV and wait for my bruises to go away. I didn't get to do that, though, because the surprise twist to this event was that as soon as I got into the car after the race, I got a text from a friend two states away imploring me to take on another new running challenge. This one was only two weeks away, and it was an all-night relay race.

Here we go again…

....

MORAL OF THE STORY:

At the end of the day, you still get the awesome stories and the same medal (or headband) as everyone else in a race, even if you're slow or don't feel hard-core enough. Or even if finishing requires someone else's hands on your rear end.

Chapter 4

THE RAGNAR RELAY

» Making Your Weekends Count «

"I thought that cheeseburger was really doing me a solid, but right now it's doing me a liquid..."

RAGNAR TEAMMATE
1:30 a.m., 18 hours into the race

While I was still finding mud in unfortunate places and counting bruises and lacerations from the Tough Mudder, I got a text from my friend Matt in Tennessee asking if I would join his team for a two-day relay race taking place in two weeks. Since I was on a runner's high from Tough Mudder, I jumped at the chance. (That's a total lie. I was exhausted and didn't want to think about running for a long time. My actual reply was, "You literally could not have picked a worse time to ask me that," and I declined. But Matt and his team kept asking me to join, so I finally relented a few days later.)

The race was called The Ragnar Relay, and it occurs in various regions across the U.S. Teams typically consist of 12 people. The routes are a total of 200 miles and take about 25 to 35 hours to complete. The race is continuous, so teams must have a runner on the course the entire time. Team members live in vans throughout the race and pass a "baton" to each other. (It was actually a slap bracelet that curled tightly around the wrist. There are portable toilets at music festivals that are more inviting to touch than that thing was after living on the sweaty arms of runners for 30+ hours. I tried not to think about it.) The baton is passed at each exchange point, until all team members cross the finish line together at the end of the journey. It's a race that combines the pure sport of running with the American childhood tradition of briefly running away from home. I can't say I wasn't intrigued.

> **PRO TIP:** Running events can offer the chance to satisfy our cravings for wild ventures. There are few occasions in adult life to go exploring for days in a van with perfect strangers, outside of being abducted.

I felt hesitant to join the team, however, because even though I'd finished several races, I was still self-conscious about my slow pace. My old fear that this race might only be for "real" runners rose up, but the team insisted they were just doing this for fun and wanted me whether I was fast or not. The teams' insistence, combined with the lure of leaving my normal routine and going on a weekend running voyage, was too strong to resist. I finally did what I always do: squeezed my eyes shut, hit the Go button, and waited to see what would happen.

The team I agreed to join included Matt—who initially invited me—and Robert, who was my youth pastor when I was in college in Tennessee. I didn't know any of the other people on our 12-person team. Former youth pastor Robert also happened to be a former Green Beret in the U.S. Army, so no matter what he told me about how "fun" and "safe" this race would be, all I could think about was the time he'd told me about eating a live rat that wandered into his cell during P.O.W. training. His threshold of "not fun" and "dangerous" was leap years away from mine.

When I joined the team, I had very few details. I didn't

know who else was coming, where we were sleeping, how many miles I would need to run—or even how much it was going to cost me. I just said yes, and tried to wait patiently for more instructions. (While I do love adventure and spontaneity, I'm also a little high-strung and controlling, so running in crazy races brings a special mix of both joy and panic for me. Even so, I've yet to regret doing any of them.) I then went through a series of alarming discoveries:

- I was asked to pick up a teammate from the airport, and I didn't know him.

- I was told I needed to figure out how to get myself and Airport Boy to West Virginia to meet the rest of the team.

- I wondered, "Why do we need to get to West Virginia if the race starts in Maryland?" and then learned that we were staying at someone's house in West Virginia the night before the race. I didn't know them, either.

- I was told that another teammate offered to pick up both me and Airport Boy and take us to West Virginia with him. And I didn't know him, either.

I finally got a call the week of the race from Airport Boy. We chatted away as if we knew each other already, because I figured everyone else on the team knew each other, and I knew Former Green Beret (FGB) Robert, so that was kind of like knowing everyone else. We ended the conversation with a plan in place for carpooling with the other guy to West Virginia.

On carpooling day, the other guy picked up Airport Boy and me, and we headed out. We made pleasant conversation about what we all do for our livings, and how I knew FGB Robert, and we got about 40 miles down the road before I finally asked how *they* knew Robert—and they didn't. I sat there with a frozen half-smile on my face, trying not to give away the fact that I had become acutely aware that I'd jumped into a car with two strangers, had given them my address, and was now being taken by them to another state.

Slightly concerned, I asked the guys how they ended up on the team, since they didn't know anyone else and didn't even know each other before this. Apparently, people can act as free agents on the Ragnar website and join teams in need of more runners. Which goes to show you: a) people love running so much they're willing to live in a van with strangers to do it, and b) you can have great running adventures even if you try something by yourself, because other runners will take you in.

> **PRO TIP:** It's not necessary to know the people around you when you're involved in a race. Runners eventually bond, because we're all testing ourselves in the same physical space. Plus everyone's gross and sweaty by the end, so that levels the playing field.

I was glad to learn I wasn't actually being kidnapped, so I turned my attention to helping us navigate to the house we were about to stay in for the night, with more people none of us knew. It was at that point that I realized FGB Robert had never given us an address. This trip was really starting out well. I called Robert and learned that he and other team members had been driving from Tennessee in one of the vans we were going to use during our race.

And that van had just broken down somewhere outside of Knoxville.

I stifled panic for the second time that day, and my car of strangers continued on to West Virginia. As we pulled up to the address Robert had given us, the homeowner walked out in curiosity. I exclaimed, "We're with Robert!" like an alien leading with "We come in peace!" It turned out the homeowner was a very nice pastor who knew FGB Robert. He told us we could all sleep in his church parsonage. Then I was told there was another girl coming to join the team and she would need to share my bed when she arrived. Sure enough, shortly after I laid down, a girl tip-toed into my room and jumped into bed with me, no words exchanged. This race was already delivering on the promise of adventure, and we hadn't even hit the start line yet.

I woke up the next morning and apparently was the last one to know about a team meeting taking place right then. I finally heard a collective "Hey, Dana!" from the living room, which coaxed me out of my room. I walked out sheepishly to see several more strangers. I waved at them and offered a feeble, "Oh hey, guys," and that's how I met the rest of my team.

The team meeting ended and everyone rushed to get in their vans and get started (at that point, we had one replacement van from Knoxville and one church van donated by the pastor we'd stayed with).

I finally got the chance to greet Matt when we all stopped to grab breakfast, and I blurted out, "I still don't know the name of the girl I slept with last night!" This undoubtedly caused even more concern among the rest of the group about just who, exactly, this crazy D.C. lady joining the team was. Shortly after that outburst, I went to the ladies' room and discovered that my shorts had been on inside-out the entire morning. And so began Race Day 1.

> **PRO TIP:** There is a place for you on race teams, even if you are slow. And don't know anyone. And can't actually dress yourself correctly.

The way Ragnar works is that each team member is assigned a number from 1 to 12, and everyone stays in that order when running. So once I finished my first leg, I'd wait for the other eleven runners to finish before I ran my second leg, and so forth. Everyone on the team ran three legs each, which varied in length and difficulty. I was assigned the least total distance, which was broken out into three legs of 5.7, 3.6, and 4.4 miles.

I was in the second van, which meant we had to wait for the six people in the first van to get through their first legs before we even started. While my van waited to receive the baton, we passed the time by checking out the other teams in the race. Runners get really into this race, sometimes wearing costumes, using noisemakers at the exchange points, and decorating their vans.

Some of our runners also passed the time by taking naps or changing into Captain America onesies before starting their legs, as one of our van-mates surprised us by quietly doing.

It was while the Captain ran his first leg that we found out our other van had lost its brakes.

This race was trying to kill us.

The team scrambled to replace yet another van, but because the race was taking place in hilly country, it was tough to get cell phone reception. We had to try various methods of texting/calling/sending carrier pigeons to communicate with each other and with the rental company. It was 6:30 pm on a Friday—and *if* we found a rental company with a van available, we would have to describe our location to them so they'd know how to find us. I began to believe we'd have to throw in the towel before I'd even run my first leg of the race.

Several phone calls and a few smoke signals later, we learned that the teammates in the broken-down van had resourcefully crammed into other peoples' vans and were heading—like fit, sweaty hitchhikers—to the next big exchange point. With the other runners taken care of for the time being, we were able to focus on finding another van. Thankfully, we secured a rental in time—and I was finally going to start my first leg.

Throughout the whole day, I'd worried that I would miss a course sign and get off track when it was my turn to carry the baton. Sure enough, as I started my first leg, I lost the course. I finally saw one girl running ahead, so I hurried to catch up. I started by confirming that she was part of the race, since the relay ran through the middles of towns so it was possible to encounter local joggers. I couldn't assume I could yell out "Hey! Ragnar!" without her Tasering me. She confirmed that she was with the race, so I started to ask which way to go. She beat me to it and asked *me* which way to go. A few steps later, a man started to pass me and I tried my question again. When I asked if he knew which direction the race was going, he replied, "No, I was following you!" We were all going to perish for lack of orienteering skills.

Instead of making peace with the fact that my demise would include starving to death in Lycra with two strangers after we failed to find our way out of a small Maryland town, I decided to comfort myself with the fact that at least I could count that first girl I passed as a kill. (A "kill" is when you pass another runner. When you get back to your team, you proudly report it and it gets marked on your van's window to intimidate other teams.)

I finally found a race sign informing me that the race course veered onto a nearby trail, and I resumed my will to live and continued my leg.

As I trotted along the serene trail, the "kill" thing started to get to me. I'd begun the leg thinking, "I just finished a Tough Mudder—I've got nothing to prove. I'm going to go slow and not worry about it." But when I spotted another runner in front of me, my inner-cage fighter screamed, "You are *mine!*"

> **PRO TIP:** Competitiveness can rise up within us at any pace. Embrace it and let it drive you forward. Just try not to yell "Kill!" when you do. Some people don't like that.

I went in for the kill and kept doing that through the whole five-plus miles of my leg. That silly little game propelled me to run a little faster than I thought I would. (I'm now considering keeping my own personal kill chart in my house and using that to make myself run faster on my own trail near home. Of course, I'll have to remind myself that no one else is playing this game with me and try not to yell "I'm coming to kill you!" when I start to pass someone. But I think I can remember not to do that.) I managed to make five kills and when I rejoined my team at the next exchange point I proudly announced, "I passed five people!" after which I had to follow it up with...

"However, ten people passed me."

My glory was short-lived. Since we kept track of *net* kills, my score at that point was minus five. And that's when I decided to follow the lead of one of my other teammates who'd finally written "pacifist" next to his name on our van window's kill tally.

After running my leg, I rode in one van while we drove to the next exchange to rejoin our other van at a high school that had opened its doors for the race. There, we could eat cafeteria food and sleep on a gym floor for a couple hours while rethinking the decision to pay for this experience. We were also offered locker room showers, for which I was grateful, even after I realized that one of the showers was broken, so I had to wait in line for one of the other three, and the one I chose tried to boil my skin. There was no way to adjust the temperature, and it was so hot I kept having to leap away to regroup before I hopped back in again and tried not to shriek. At one point I started giggling at how absurd the whole scene was. I overheard a group of other runners waiting in line comment that, "This process would work better if people got in and out more quickly. You can't ponder life in there."

I took pleasure in thinking about those girls getting

scalded themselves.

I finally finished my torture shower, and our van eventually hit the road again. It was time for my dreaded night run. I was nervous about the night run because I had heard that I might be completely alone. I feared a) getting lost again and/or b) getting picked up by a van full of strangers that wasn't part of the race.

Thankfully, my night leg was full of other runners, so I was never out of sight of another bobbing headlamp. It was like running with a bunch of giant fireflies and actually made a nice, if surreal, experience. We ran through a quiet subdivision and then past long stretches of corn fields. All the while, the other vans would drive past, occasionally yelling out encouragement. One of the other faceless fireflies flittered up beside me as we were nearing the next exchange and yelled out, "Run towards the liiiiight!" I laughed and obeyed his order, following the light right back to my van.

Somewhere around 12:30 a.m., we pulled into an exchange at a cow farm that was serving cheeseburgers. Most of my teammates ordered burgers while we waited for our next runner to come in. People were eating, even though it was 12:30 a.m. and we had just eaten spaghetti at the high school a couple hours before. As we stood in line, we got alternating whiffs of live cattle and cooked hamburger, giving us the full Circle of Life to ponder. There was very little that could make us uncomfortable by that point.

Reaching the level of apathy where one can consume an animal right in front of its family members was one of the special gifts of this race.

The whole event was disorienting, in part because we lacked sleep and proper nutrition. We lost track of time, and lost the ability to care, so the relay felt like one really long, poorly lived day.

Our tired minds brought about interesting conversations. When my van passed a male runner wearing gold lamé shorts and a superhero sign painted on his bare chest, Captain America opened the van door and yelled out: "I like yer britches!" in his southern accent. The other people in my van noted that the poor guy in the shorts would probably have to look up the term "britches" in the Urban Dictionary. "Or the *Rural* Dictionary…" mumbled another teammate, as we all chuckled before resuming our exhausted blank stares out the windows.

My team continued to become increasingly delirious until the sun came up. We greeted the new day with, you guessed it—more running! By that point, we had wound our way back into D.C., so I was feeling more comfortable. The last leg I had to do was on a portion of my regular running trail, so at least if I got lost again, I could just give up and walk home.

As we entered D.C., we pulled into an exchange that was serving pancakes. There were runners lying on the ground, desperately trying to get a little more sleep wherever they could. Again, I questioned our judgment in paying to do this.

After wiping pancake syrup off ourselves, we continued on to finish the last few legs of the race—and that was when we realized we were completely out of water. I'm never running away with these people again.

I could've dealt without water at that point, since I *only* had a 4.4-mile leg left, and after running so much already, four miles seemed hardly significant. However, some of my teammates had longer legs left to run. To make things even more exciting, the only other female runner on our team was *pregnant.* She'd found out right before we started the race, and ran with our crazy group anyway.

> **PRO TIP:** if you need ammunition against excuses to not run a race, know that someone, somewhere, is probably running a 200-mile relay with another human inside her body. That means you can get through it, too.

I took it upon myself to find us all more water. I started with the team nearest us, whose van was painted with the words "Creepy Van Running Club" on the front, and "Cute Puppies!" and "Free Candy!" on either side. I attempted to be cute, too, and asked, "I don't need candy, but would you possibly have a bottle of water you'd let me have?" I batted my eyelashes. They said no.

Jerks. You'll never kidnap people with that attitude!

I persevered and stalked another van and found success. The team in that van embodied the runner community spirit I love. They wouldn't let me take only one bottle, but gave me an entire jug of water. I triumphantly took my spoils back to our van and we drove off yet again. Finally, it was time to complete my last leg. I held out my wrist for the baton bracelet, tried not to flinch from how obviously germ-infested it was by then, and off I went.

I finished my leg of the race and handed off the baton to FGB Robert, who would carry it to the end. My van drove to the finish, where my teammates and I heaved our sore, tired bodies out onto the road one last time. We hobbled to gather around Robert as he approached the end, all trotting across the finish line together, no longer sure what time—or day—it was, but sure we would proudly tell our grandkids about this someday.

. . . .

MORAL OF THE STORY:

Shaking up your daily routine with a crazy race adventure makes hitting the pavement time and time again during training all worth it. In races—as in life—the prize is in the journey. The finish line is nice, but getting there is half the fun. Even when your van smells.

Chapter 5

RUNNING FOR BOSTON: THE RUN NOW RELAY

» Six Days of Running for a Cause «

"… divide the race into thirds. Run the first part with your head, the middle part with your person-ality, and the last part with your heart."

MIKE FANELLI, RUNNING CLUB COACH

On April 15, 2013, tragedy struck the ultimate running event: the Boston Marathon.

If you're part of the running community, Boston holds a special place in your heart. The marathon there is the capstone event for runners. The bombs that went off on April 15, 2013, struck our fellow runners and the supporters who cheer us along. On the day of the attack, I couldn't focus on my meeting at work and found myself nearly in tears, muttering, "They got their legs. This is a running event and they got their legs." I immediately joined every "response run" I found around D.C. People gathered to run together to prove that we weren't afraid, and to stand in solidarity with the sport and with the community that means so much to us.

A few months after the Boston Marathon attack, I heard from my Tennessee runner friends again, some of the same people I ran Ragnar with. They too felt like they had to do something in response to Boston. They started formulating a plan to raise money for the victims, then decided to physically deliver the check themselves by running from Tennessee to Boston in a 1000-mile relay, arriving in time for the Boston Marathon in 2014. They called it The Run Now Relay, and they asked if I wanted to join. It seemed crazy to run a relay five times the length of Ragnar, but how could I say no?

I was amazed by the efforts of my friends to come up with such a crazy race, then build it out and train to run it over the next several months, on top of their regular jobs and family duties.

The team ultimately included 26 runners who would run a total of 1,075 contiguous miles through seven states in eight days. An engineer on the team created the route, and the operation included volunteer drivers; a mobile command center in the form of a semi-truck; a media team to help raise awareness and money; and countless sponsors donating food, race shirts, and hotel rooms along the way. Everyone pulled together to make the race happen, embodying the humanitarianism and determination I've come to love in the running community as a whole.

> **PRO TIP:** Another reason to love runners is their drive and compassion. Several people who were able to finish the Boston Marathon on the day of the bombings then ran several more blocks to donate blood to the victims at the nearest hospital. How can you not love a community made up of people like that?

While the cause we would run the Run Now Relay to benefit was a serious one, the race itself—like most others I've been involved in—would result in many funny moments. The first one was when I agreed to join and found myself, yet again, saying yes before fully understanding the commitment. My friend Matt originally invited me in July of 2013. Here's a timeline of the events that ensued:

July 19, 2013—Nearly a year before the relay. Matt: "Would you be interested in flying to Tennessee and running the entire route with us?"

I decide I can't take that much time off work, but I could serve as a half member of the team, joining them for the second 500 miles of the journey, from D.C. to Boston.

January 23, 2014. I discreetly leave my desk to take a selfie in the bathroom at work in order to have a photo for the official team website. I am now committed.

Hence began a tornado of relay emails, group texts, instructions, requests, media inquiries, preparations, and out-of-office requests to my bosses that simply read "Dana Out: Running from here to Boston." But I still didn't know many details. I proceeded to try to walk the line between being cool and being a Type A personality who needs details like I need oxygen. I was partially successful.

February 4, 2014—Two months before the relay. Me: "Hey Matt! I just realized I never asked how long you will need me to run in the relay. I just blindly said yes, haha." ("Haha" = The universal way to conceal the sheer panic behind your actual message.) "Do you know how far I'll be running each day? No worries if not..."

Matt: "Yes, you should probably have asked before now. We have you down for 25 miles per day."

Haha. Good thing he's kidding. I think.

The weeks went on and there was discussion about what the team members needed to bring to stay fed, hydrated, seen in the dark, and protected from vicious dogs. There was talk of bringing firearms, which are frowned upon in D.C., and I pictured us all getting thrown in jail before I started my first leg. There were repeated reminders that this was "an adventure" and we all needed to "be flexible." I kept flashing back to the Ragnar, where all of our vehicles broke down and we were reduced to disoriented shells of our former selves, eating cattle at two in the morning because we weren't sure what time it was or when we would be able to eat next.

March 12, 2014–One month before the race. Matt, casually: "We don't have confirmations on hotel rooms yet, so sleeping arrangements are going to be hit and miss at times!"

I like adventure. I like adventure. I like adventure.

The team was separated into different vehicle groups called *flights*, and everyone was assigned to one the week before the race. We had five flights total. Each flight would need to collectively run 30 miles on each leg of the race. Like the Ragnar race, the legs were contiguous, so it was possible for one flight to have a leg that started at 1:00 a.m. then another at 8:00 p.m. that night. Legs might go through farmland in Delaware, or through downtown Manhattan. I missed the meeting where flights were assigned, so I was still clueless about everything until right before the race started.

April 9, 2014—One week out. Me, still trying to sound nonchalant: "I'd love to know what my legs are if you have a chance to send them."

April 14, 2014—Two days before I jump into one of the race vehicles. Me: "Matt, can you send me my leg info?"

I never got a reply.

I did finally get word that I'd be in Matt's flight.

After the team as a whole did a ceremonial run with D.C. running groups along the National Mall, I jumped into my race vehicle to head to Baltimore, where a hotel was waiting for us so we could try to get some sleep. It was 5:30 p.m.

Because the team had been running for a few days already by the time I joined them, people were on erratic schedules that revolved around two main questions: a) "Am I about to run?" and, if the answer was no, b) "Is that a surface? Then I'm sleeping on it." To force my body to jump into that erratic rhythm too, I set my alarm in Baltimore to wake me up at 2:17 a.m. I had officially joined the craziness.

Accommodations for the relay ranged from actual hotels to the floor of a church to the bunk beds inside the traveling command center, which broke down a few times. Additionally, there was never a time block that felt longer than four hours in which to sleep anyway, given our running schedule. Many times, team members would check in and check out of a hotel the same day, passing their keys off to the flights that came in behind them—and they lived like that for six days straight. Ladies and gentlemen, I give you: runners.

My vehicle was Flight Three, which meant our legs always started once everyone in Flight Two finished. The entire team's progress was tracked through a GPS device we lovingly referred to as "GPSy" (pronounced "gypsy," and referred to as "her"), which each runner handed off to the next. Carrying GPSy as we ran enabled supporters to track where the team was in real time. (This system worked well, unless someone, say, forgot they had GPSy after they ran, then walked around with her on in an IKEA store; or if, say, someone dropped and killed her, causing the team to go dark for a bit while finding a replacement. All hypothetical situations, of course.)

We left our hotel in Baltimore around 3:00 a.m. to meet Flight Two for the GPSy hand off. Our first runner of the day was a guy we'd dubbed The Race Horse, as he had committed to run a marathon a day through the entire six-day relay, *before* he went on to finish the Boston Marathon—*in less than half the time it had taken me to finish my marathon.* He literally ran across the entire state of Delaware for us. He was a machine. After getting hold of GPSy, he effortlessly glided away from us at a ridiculous speed.

It really was beautiful to watch him. It was like he was sprinting, but he held that pace for 26 miles, looking at ease the entire time. We'd call him during his legs to check in and he'd sound like he was reclined on a sofa somewhere. I would've hated him had he not been so nice.

> **PRO TIP:** While I consider myself a proud ambassador of slow runners, I will say it is pretty amazing to watch a naturally fast runner in action. It's like watching a cheetah. Or the gazelle running for its life from the cheetah—without the obvious panic and unsightly death that follows.

Our journey after we launched The Race Horse felt very similar to Ragnar: disorienting. I never knew who was running, which flight was next, what state we were in, etc. It was a constant, confusing churn of relayers all over the East Coast. Additionally, we had a travelling documentary team filming the race. We were also contacting local media along the route, so team members were constantly giving interviews at strange hours. I can't imagine what it's like for famous rock stars who live that kind of schedule every day, but I can say I'm not surprised that they start using cocaine.

Our team included some people with strong personalities, which resulted in amusing, sleep-deprived antics. Former Green Beret Robert from my Ragnar team was in another flight on this run and he began photographing his overenthusiastic face next to the defenseless head of anyone who fell asleep in his van, then posting the photos on social media. Also, at one point, the driver of my flight was found chasing another runner down the road with a dead squirrel he'd found. Maybe endorphins do more than make you happy—maybe they block the neurons that transmit maturity.

Since the flights were leap-frogging each other, I really didn't see a lot of my teammates in person. And since only one vehicle had runners on the road at any given time, the other flights had time to kill before they ran again. So I'd see group text messages where one flight would be telling the next what mile they were on, while another flight exclaimed they'd found an outlet mall in Jersey, while another would announce they were heading out to get a Geno's Cheesesteak in Philly.

Sometimes we wouldn't realize what state another flight was in until we saw a reporter interviewing them for the news. Other times we'd find out a flight was in trouble only after a message popped up on our cell phone screens stating something like "Flight 2: Minor delay ..." with a photo attached of a police car in their rearview mirror. When we did run into other flights, we'd all quickly swap tales and learn things. Like the fact that one of the vehicles broke down right before their runner was stopped by police, who then questioned him as to why he was trying to run on the Jersey Turnpike. That runner's phone battery died at that exact moment, and I never even heard how he made it back to safety. We'd all end conversations mid-story to rush off to sleep somewhere or to jump back in our vehicles to hit the road again. But no one ever had a negative attitude. Not even the teammate who accidentally peed in her pants during her leg when she couldn't find a restroom, earning her the nickname Pee Wee.

> **PRO TIP:** Another reward of the running community: Most runners have experienced something gross like toenails falling off or snot rockets shooting out of their nose, so they tend to be a less judgmental group of people than most.

We'd all end up with nicknames before the relay was over. Like "Wrong Way EK" for our teammate whose initials were EK and who had a knack for always taking incorrect turns. Or "Puddles," the nickname for our leader Matt, who kept getting emotional during the journey. (My nickname ended up being "Wedge," after I accidentally got a race vehicle stuck in a parking garage, which technically happened after the relay was over, so I think that it should be forgotten for lack of relevancy, but no one else agrees.)

The team's positive attitude was especially admirable given that members encountered everything from freezing temperatures to 80-degree weather, massive hills, and running right next to speeding traffic. I did worry a little about how the group would fare running through Philadelphia or Manhattan at all hours of the night, but thankfully everyone came through unscathed. And the support that built around the relay made it all feel worth it. Since our vehicles had donation information painted on them, people would honk or send us Twitter messages—some even came up to us to donate money on the spot. It was incredible.

The camaraderie in the flights became intense. Some teammates would run together just for each other's company or to get more miles in (we had some ultra-marathoners on the team who were training for their next races, but we also had novice runners, so it was a nice mix). I was with two other runners on my first six-mile leg, rather than running that leg alone—thankfully, because about two miles in I experienced my first ever debilitating calf cramp.

In all my years of running, I'd never been completely stopped by a cramp like that. My calf muscle seized up and would not release. I ended up having to jump back in the van, dejected, while my teammates continued without me. The Race Horse gave me tips on relieving it, but when we got out to eat a little while later, I could still barely walk. Thankfully, after a short "night's sleep" in the middle of the day, massages, and lots of prayer, I was able to run again by the time GPSy came back around to my hands. At that point, we were about to enter New York City—in the middle of the night.

I think everyone was a little nervous about the New York City night run. I ran with the other female in my flight and we stayed close to the vehicle for safety in the more desolate areas. We were all relieved when we finally neared Times Square, right before sunrise. At that point, there was no opportunity for sleep because the team was about to be on *Good Morning America*. (Trust me, the *best* time to be on national television is when you're drenched in sweat, haven't slept all night, and are wearing your "I will never be asked out in this" running beanie.) Even as most of the team was being taped for the segment, we still had one flight on the road, because the race went on, no matter what.

After the *Good Morning America* interview, we headed out again. My van got GPSy somewhere in Connecticut. We were on our last leg. I was running the flight's final six miles alone, proudly carrying GPSy one last time. Around 10:30 p.m., I was trotting along on a fairly untraveled road, with our van slightly ahead of me, when all of a sudden a big waba truck came up behind me. Its driver did not seem friendly. (Waba [*WAH-buh*] truck: Me and my southern friend's pet name for those large, jacked-up trucks, typically driven in rural areas. Accessories may include giant chrome exhaust pipes, enormous tires, and engines that idle loudly, making a *waba waba* noise. Waba trucks are revved strategically, particularly during mating season or to display the driver's obvious manliness.)

The truck crept slowly past me, whipped a U-turn to come back, pulled up next to me, and started revving the motor. I anxiously looked up toward my van as the waba truck continued to creep along near me. I jogged a little faster, picturing a drunken redneck behind the wheel with a shotgun, and the truck started to slowly pass yet again as the driver stared at me. That was when I uncontrollably channeled Tony Soprano. I raised my hands, shrugged my shoulders violently at the driver and yelled, "*What?!*" (Shortly after that, it occurred to me that it was possible this guy was only trying to donate money, which would have been really awkward. But he wasn't. He continued to be creepy.)

I kept my eye on my van and continued on. Then, all of a sudden, the flight van door opened and out leapt... The Race Horse.

The Race Horse didn't even wait for the van to come to a stop before he flew out and started jogging by my side. He looked around, *picked up a stick,* and started running alongside me, weapon in hand, staring menacingly toward the truck, daring it to do anything. The truck finally drove off. And even though the whole experience rattled me, it was worth it just to be able to say: *I. Ran. With. The Race Horse!* (It totally still counts, even if my running pace is more like his walking pace. If he had broken an ankle.)

> **PRO TIP:** Even though my pace was much slower and I didn't log as many miles, my runs were just as celebrated by our team as The Race Horse's runs. That is how the running community is: People celebrate each other's personal wins, at every level.

After I ran my leg, we checked into our hotel near Boston. In the morning, we saw other flight members downstairs eating breakfast so we started comparing stories from the road again. People had shifted around and swapped legs occasionally, so it was fun to hear what everyone had ended up logging by the end. I heard someone proudly announce that his flight-mate ran 20 miles the day before. "The longest he'd ever run before that was eight miles—and that was Tuesday!" The journey had definitely pushed us all in new ways.

We got back on the road and headed toward the start line for the Boston Marathon, which would be the finish line for our relay. We still had one flight on the road, and the plan was to have the entire team link up with the last runner and run together to finish the relay as one.

Everyone was tired, but when our last runner came into view, we all got a shot of adrenaline and took off towards the line together. It was emotional, to say the least. We ended up raising more than $65,000, and had earned the tagline "Boston Strong, Tennessee Tough."

The next day, several of the team members headed back to their families, while the rest of us stayed to cheer on our teammates who were running the Boston Marathon. (Besides The Race Horse, who qualified to run the Boston Marathon, our team received charity bibs for three other members to run the prestigious race *after* they'd run all the way there from several states away. One of them was in his 50s. Runners–gotta love 'em.)

How do I explain watching the Boston Marathon? I've run in dozens of races through the years, including finishing my own marathon. I know what it feels like to be cheered on and encouraged by strangers when you need it. But I felt new levels of emotion while I stood on the sideline and cheered on other runners, other strangers, and saw the looks of appreciation on their tired faces.

I started watching from the finish line with some friends from the relay and saw Meb Keflezighi win. Then, a little while later, I watched our own Race Horse finish. It was exhilarating to be at the finish, but it was even more poignant when we moved back a bit and stood along the road at the second to last turn the runners make: Hereford. There's a famous phrase that anyone involved with the Boston Marathon knows: *Right on Hereford, left on Boylston*. Those are the final directions before you see the finish line. Once you reach that point, you know you're in the home stretch. I watched multiple runners start to cry as soon as they hit that turn.

We saw people wearing shirts noting how far the wearer got in 2013 before the bombs went off. We saw so much determination to finish what had been started the year before. We saw men pushing sons in wheelchairs, people running alongside blind runners, people running in memory of others, firefighters, National Guardsmen. Something came over me in the midst of screaming "You got this!!!!" to people I'll never actually meet and waving my cowbell like I was possessed, and I spontaneously burst into tears.

> **PRO TIP:** Races are a microcosm of life. When you see someone overcome obstacles to reach their race goal, it's like watching a victory for the human race in general. Bring tissues.

We watched as the other three of our Run Now Relay runners, including my friend and our leader Matt, rounded that last corner. Predictably, Matt turned into puddles when he saw us. I tear up to this day just thinking of it.

Before I headed to the airport, I visited the post-race banquet to congratulate our runners. When the plane was being boarded, anyone who had run the Boston Marathon was allowed to board first. Clearly, this whole city revered their marathon, and after finally watching it in person, I understood why. I saw such resilience in that city, and in the marathon runners and supporters. It made me fall in love with running all over again.

....

MORAL OF THE STORY:

If you need to renew your faith in humanity, watch a marathon. Or, better yet, run in a challenging race or relay with other people. The stuff we're made of that rises to the surface during such times makes all the effort worth it.

Chapter 6

CROSS-TRAINING
» Running Side Dishes «

"I have to exercise in the morning before my brain figures out what I'm doing."

MARSHA DOBLE

Runners' blogs and fitness magazines contain many tips on how to improve form or increase strength and speed, but sometimes what I really need is the motivation to keep going when I'd much rather be reclined in front of a *Real Housewives* marathon, my face covered in Cheetos dust and resignation.

Staring at a photo of a toned runner who I want to look like only takes me so far before I give up and convince myself that life can be just as fulfilling in a pudgy and breathless body. Thankfully, along the way, I've stumbled upon my own personal tricks for staying motivated. I still don't resemble the fitness magazine cover girls, but I've managed to stay in decent shape, enough to continue running races with the middle-to-back-of-the-pack folk.

One of my big motivators is fun. If something isn't enjoyable, I typically don't see the point in doing it. I also need variety. Boredom has always been one of my greatest fears, so much so that as a child I would pack 10 different toys when I went to Grandma's house, just in case I felt the urge to read a book, then play Go Fish, then color a picture, then create a Care Bear vs. My Little Pony epic battle, all within the first hour. *I can't just play with Barbies all* day, *Mom. Do you want me to die?*

Thankfully, to be a good runner you need to do more than run. You also need to cross-train, which shakes things up.

"Cross-training: training in two or more sports in order to improve fitness and performance, especially in a main sport."

— *Oxford Dictionary.*

I play fast and loose with the word *sport* in that definition. Here is a list of ways I've cross-trained (which are really just ways I keep exercising when I'm not running, or things I do that resemble exercise when I don't really feel like exercising):

Zumba. The class where you can feel like Shakira until you accidentally glance in the mirror and realize you look more like a baby deer trying to salsa dance.

Yoga. Where everyone's a calm adult until someone accidentally passes gas in Tree Pose.

Rowing. I have nothing funny to say about rowing because this sport is no joke and will use muscles you never knew you had, while making you so exhausted you actually nap after practice and you *never nap.* (Ok I lied, there is one funny thing about rowing and that was when my friend and I had to sit through the safety video where the symptoms of hypothermia were explained, in case we ever fell out of the boat in frigid waters. One symptom? "Apathy." My friend has wondered daily if she is hypothermic at work ever since.)

Indoor climbing. I'm scared of ~~heights~~ equipment and/or human failure, so this is always a particularly masochistic type of exercise for me. I've had moments of panic 40 feet in the air, when I've yelled, "TAKE! *Taaaaaaake!!!*" at the poor guy belaying me below, a guy who'd already taken all the slack humanly possible out of the rope holding me, and I still felt too vulnerable. Climbing is a good workout for different parts of the body used for running, though. And if nothing else, doing it makes me love running more, merely for the fact that running doesn't require me to wear a diaper-like harness—unless I want to.

Trapeze. *Yes.* My philosophy in life is pretty much summed up as: Do everything you possibly can, even if it scares you. So, in spite of my fear of heights, I have tried the trapeze, too. It turned out to be incredibly fun and empowering. Judging from my soreness the next day, it was also very good for building a strong core. Moreover, my instructors wore tight pants and no shirts and I am now considering joining a dating site for circus staff.

Moon Bouncing. Ok, this one isn't actually a regular sport that I do—nor is it an official sport at all—but I have adult friends who rent those inflatable bounce house things for parties. I've not only jumped in them (which totally counts as a workout), but I've taken part in an original game called Deflate Escape. Deflate Escape was created when my friend Ryan realized we could pull the plug on the moon bounce house, which would begin to deflate it, and then everyone inside could attack each other while trying to escape out the hatch on top before we all suffocated. It was very cutthroat, so I consider that cross-training for life in general.

> **PRO TIP:** A perk of being a non-competitive runner is that you don't have to take cross-training terribly seriously unless you want to. Just do something besides running, call it cross-training, and then call it a day.

Spin class. Spinning—riding a stationary bicycle—is one of my favorite things to do, and not only because I had an instructor at Gold's Gym who used to get so excited in spin class that he would yell at all of us as we pedaled furiously, "*Give Daddy what he wants!*" (He was later fired, I heard. I guess I can understand why.) Something comes over everyone when they enter a spin room. Even highly intelligent people get sucked in and blindly follow an instructor's orders to "Get up that hill!" or "Race!"— even though at the beginning of the class we all knew we were getting on bikes that couldn't actually go anywhere. It's like we turn into trusting dogs whose owners tease by making a throwing motion – but not actually throwing anything. *Is that a hill? Is it?! Are we coming up on a hill!!? Because I'm totally pedaling harder if we're coming up on a hill!!* Plus, with the dim lights and pumping music, it feels like what I imagine a rave must feel like, except no one is on drugs (except maybe those instructors who see imaginary hills ahead).

Boot Camp Classes. I don't know the actual definition for what a boot camp workout is, but I've taken classes called boot camps in which we've done everything from running around with sand bags over our shoulders to hitting a tractor tire with a sledge hammer. The workouts feel primal and oddly satisfying. Plus, if I'm ever in a situation where I have to do 20 burpees (a sadistic jump/push-up move) or someone will kill one of my family members, I'm now totally prepared to be the hero.

CrossFit. CrossFit is the sport where, according to one of my friends, "You work out one hour, then spend the next 23 hours talking about it." I had heard rumors from several people that CrossFit was cult-like and all-consuming, and that it pushed people so hard they injured themselves. I was hesitant, but one of my friends and running partners, Adam, convinced me to try it anyway. It was also the trendy thing to do at that point, so of course I considered it even if it promised to be painful (see Chapter One re: drugless births and my FOMO condition). Having successfully finished tough races, I had built up enough confidence to try other new things, so I proceeded to my first CrossFit experience.

I headed out to meet Adam for class and found him inside a mixed martial arts (MMA) gym. Not only was I about to potentially join the CrossFit cult, but before I even got to the CrossFit part of the gym, I had to push past bloodthirsty fighters waiting to jump into the ring. The smell alone in the MMA part of the gym should've been enough to make me defect immediately.

Adam and I got to the CrossFit area and it was packed. Heavy metal music blared, bodies all over the room intermingled with equipment I'd never seen before, people yelled encouragement to others who were pumping some of the biggest weights I'd ever seen. Everyone *did* seem a little obsessed. I concentrated on not allowing my face to show fear as I thought, *Yep, this is definitely a cult.* I felt so grateful that Adam was with me, and then, right off the bat, the class instructors split us up. *This is how they get us. They're separating me from my herd.*

They put me with three other ladies who were also new. We started the class by jogging outside, after which I was winded and worried. *Maybe I should stick with running a little while longer before trying a new sport, because clearly I haven't mastered running yet.* Then we walked over to barbell racks where we were told to get up under a barbell, do one rep of a shoulder press, then put the barbell back on the rack. We were to keep doing that, increasing the weight, until we "failed," meaning we literally couldn't push the weight all the way up and lock our arms anymore.

I saw men raising weights entirely too big to be realistic, and then start violently shaking, nearing collapse, before hurling the barbell down far too close to me for comfort. I thought about how stupid all of this was. *Why are we picking things up? What is this proving?* And then I discovered I was able to lift more weight than half my group and I immediately started feeling that same feeling I'd had during the Ragnar Relay when I saw a potential kill: *a thirst for blood.* I heard myself beg my instructor to allow me to try just one more rep with heavier weights. *They didn't even have to bite my neck. I'm willingly turning myself*

*into a CrossFit vampire not ten minutes into class. What is
wrong with me? Do they pump addiction through the air
vents here? No wonder people push themselves so hard they
get injured all the time.*

> **PRO TIP:** Strength training with weights really
> does improve running. Maybe start in a less
> intense atmosphere though, one where you
> won't immediately feel like channeling a
> WWE wrestler and start beating your chest,
> yelling "I will destroy you, barbell!!!"

We moved onto the WOD. (WOD means Workout of
the Day—cult speak, clearly. I assumed I'd get a tear-stain
tattoo on my cheek if I ever completed one successfully,
or at least some kind of honor patch on the back brace I'd
inevitably end up in). The WOD was called *Fran*, and I
got about three different explanations for why WODs are
named after people, so I'm just going to believe that they
are named after people who died attempting them.

During the WOD, my group ended up lying on the floor
under some contraption. Rings had been suspended,
reaching almost to the ground. We were to grab the rings,
keep our bodies straight, our feet on the floor, and hoist
our upper bodies up. Because the class was so packed, we
ended up smooshed against some guys doing a different
workout close by. One of them started performing a type
of pull-up move that I'd never seen before, right above

us. It was as if he was doing The Worm in mid-air. It's apparently called a Kipping Pull-Up, and is a variation that's designed to generate momentum for the pull-up through a violent jerking motion done with the whole body. These convulsions were happening right over our heads.

I watched indignantly as the pull-up guy nearly kicked my partner in the face while she was attempting the WOD ring pull-up thingy. But... I had to admit, pull-up guy was *fit*. And shirtless. I finally gave up being coy and blatantly stared at him, analyzing all the body art he had on his torso. *I'm sorry, if you don't want to be unabashedly gawked at, don't look that good shirtless. It's a simple rule.*

At that mesmerizing moment, I may have come close to becoming a CrossFit convert.

Then it was my turn to lie on the floor and attempt to pull myself up on those stupid rings, and I snapped back to my senses. I foolishly asked the instructor about "proper form" for the ring exercise. I'm surprised he didn't laugh right in my face, because he knew what was about to happen. By my third rep, I was doing any kind of motion I could to get my body anywhere near off the floor and couldn't have cared less about proper form. You know how children who don't want to move will just go limp? You try to pull them up off the carpet but their heads lay there at an awkward angle while you tug at their arms from above? That's pretty much the "form" I had by the end of my turn of holding on to those rings.

At some point during my last rep, my contact lens slipped off my eye. *Even my eyeballs are working in this class.* I had to walk back out past the MMA testosterone ring to get to the ladies' room to fix it, and that's when I realized I could no longer straighten my arms. I was walking like a T-Rex and couldn't help it.

I won't be joining a CrossFit gym anytime soon.

Sure, I'm glad I "get" the CrossFit culture a little bit now, and I did enjoy it, but I think if I decide to join a fitness cult, I'll look for one whose members are devoted to time in the steam room, or the juice bar. I'll look for more of a spa cult, really. Until I find one of those, I'll stick to my running and less intense forms of cross-training. (Please don't take offense, CrossFitters, but it just wasn't my thing. Don't kill me. Even though you totally can, with your bare hands.)

PRO TIP: Honestly, I think biking and swimming are solid enough choices for legitimate cross-training activities. Of course, then you run the risk of getting sucked into the triathlon world. I assume the inhabitants of that world are just as crazy as runners, so maybe master one addiction at a time.

Classes at my gym, on the other hand, can be a nice cross-training activity because a) they are not CrossFit, and b) it's really nice to let go and shirk the responsibility of whipping myself into shape. When I'm running, I control how hard I push myself or how far I go. That's a lot of pressure. I'd rather blame a class instructor when my thighs still touch each other, because obviously she didn't push me hard enough, and that's her fault. Classes are also preferable because sometimes it's nice to have someone bear witness to how hard I'm sweating. Otherwise, it's like working out and not posting it on social media. *Did it really happen if no one knows it happened?*

Actually, posting on social media is another trick I sometimes use to keep myself running. I don't do it often, but every now and then I make it public that I'm going for a run. That way, I've committed myself a little more. I have to run, then, for pride's sake. Plus, I use a running app where I hear applause in my headphones every time someone "likes" my status, so that's fun. When I do a particularly good job of running in a week, that app also gives me messages from professional athletes. On days when I don't feel like running, I might do it anyway just to hear Tim Tebow tell me he's proud of me. Apps like that should exist for other things in life. I'd like to have Bradley Cooper give me a high five whenever I send an especially well-crafted email, or when I use restraint and resist the urge to yell, "*Pick a lane, Buddy!*" at the car in front of me in city traffic. Really, I'd like to have Bradley Cooper touch my hand in general, for any reason.

Applause and celebrity affirmation aren't the only things

running apps offer. Many of them employ the concept of gamification, where elements of game-playing are added to encourage users to engage with the app. As runners, for instance, we can now use an app to compare our time or distance stats to other people's. We can also use an app to chart our own progress. This is the same concept used by charity fundraisers when they display a thermometer-type graphic to show a rise in donations. We're wired to be a little competitive, so it's rewarding to have some way of displaying the score.

Another app I use donates money to my charity of choice whenever I log so many miles. That, too, nudges me to get active on days when I don't really feel like it. It's like I'm getting paid to move, so I *have* to move because I'm pretty cheap and hate leaving money on the table.

> **PRO TIP:** There are tons of ways to get yourself moving that are basically the equivalent of making an airplane noise to fly mashed-up vegetables into a child's mouth. Find whatever trick works for you to get you to do your workouts.

Sometimes it's not even running, but walking, that will bump up the stats on fitness apps, so they can also be used for cross-training—if you consider walking cross-training, and of course I do. I find myself walking more, instead of driving, so I can see the dollar sign rise on my charity app or so I can hear Serena Williams tell me I put in more work this week than last. Multi-tasking exercise and transporting myself to destinations is really important, because sometimes there isn't time to work *and* socialize *and* exercise, which is how I've ended up jogging while holding a coffee cup instead of a water bottle (because I needed a refill *and* I needed to workout), or walking two miles with a backpack full of cotija cheese and four ears of corn because I needed to have dinner at a friend's house *and* I needed to work out *and* Mexican corn doesn't just make itself.

There are other fun ways I've found to fit exercise into my schedule. Sometimes I'll sit on a stability ball instead of a chair at my desk. Doing that works your core *and* allows you to bop up and down while on boring webinars (word to the wise—just remember to turn off your webcam). Sometimes I'll ask friends to meet me for paddle boarding instead of dinner. Even if they refuse, it can be fun to be *that* friend, the one who makes everyone else feel like they aren't working hard enough at their fitness levels. It's a win-win, really.

MORAL OF THE STORY:

One way to stay in racing shape is to make cross-training fun—by any means necessary. Trick yourself, find an overzealous spin instructor, or attend a class that allows you to stare at shirtless men—you'll probably see me there too.

Chapter 7

RACES
» Making Fun Mandatory «

"The reason we race isn't so much to beat each other, but to be with each other."

CHRISTOPHER MCDOUGALL, *BORN TO RUN*

One way I stay in my relationship with running is by occasionally signing up for races that don't give me the option to *not* have fun. Races like one called Wipeout, where I ran a 5K that included amusing obstacles like giant slides and foamy chutes that racers had to glide through between miles. I'd pretty much commit to anything for a little while longer if it promised my inner child a reward. (I should've given that pointer to some of my ex-boyfriends before they became exes. I would have been more reluctant to break up with them had they regularly plunked a water slide or a foam pit in front of me to play with. And the next time my wireless carrier asks me to renew my contract, I should probably ask what the odds are of being pushed on a swing or thrown into a ball pit before signing.)

In addition to running races with carnivalesque obstacles, I've completed a couple of night runs where everyone wore glow sticks. Honestly, it's impossible to only run during these races. I inevitably skip, leap, reenact the "Gangnam Style" video, or swing a glow stick over my head like a lasso, because how can you not twirl away stress with abandon when it's too dark for people to recognize your face? Sometimes runners get so into it that they miss a couple turns and accidentally run even longer than required. At least I've heard that can happen.

I've also run a race that included chocolate handouts at the aid stop and the presentation of a Tiffany's necklace. *Yes.* The Nike Women's Half Marathon is an amazing race geared toward females, and it was held in D.C. in 2014. Not only did they pump me up by projecting my name next to encouragement on giant screens along the course, they also offered chocolate at one of the aid stations, and the race medal was an actual Tiffany's necklace that was handed out by firemen wearing tuxedos. At the time of the race, I had another terrible calf cramp and was one week away from major surgery for a giant benign tumor in my abdomen, but I was not about to be deterred. There is nothing more fun than dapper emergency responders offering luxury jewelry. *Nothing.*

> **PRO TIP:** If you need a reason to train for a race, find a race that offers the chance to goof off, eat candy, or play with nice jewelry. Basically anything your mom told you not to do as a child–except hit your sibling. There are no races that allow you to do that. Yet.

I've also run races where everyone promised to be there with bells on—literally. There's a race in D.C. called the Jingle All the Way 8K. My friend Rebekah convinced me to do it a few years ago. I figured if they really tied jingle bells to everyone's shoes, it was either going to be fun or I was going to lose my hearing. Either way, it'd be a new experience.

The start line for Jingle All the Way was fantastic, because many people wore costumes. Rebekah and I took off and were immediately passed by several characters. First, Santa and his reindeer (runners were tied together, with one dressed like Santa in the back and the rest of the runners dressed like reindeer in front of him), which was humbling since that was a group of people *tied together* and they *still* passed us.

A few steps later, we were passed by the entire Nativity scene.

The Nativity group was awesome. The Wise Men wore head scarves that flapped in the breeze and they carried boxes representing their gifts. An actual baby played Baby Jesus, and he rode along in a jogging stroller. The star had a sign on her back saying, "Follow me!" And I did, until the star stole the stuffed sheep one of the shepherds was holding, causing the shepherd to chase her through the crowd and leave me in their dust.

> **PRO TIP:** Find ways to enjoy yourself in a race, even if that entails stealing someone else's sheep.

Later in the race, I heard a bunch of voices behind me and turned to find a pack of Christmas... *bunnies?* A group of people had, inexplicably, dressed as pink bunnies, which made no sense in a Christmas race, but not a lot makes sense in a race designed to fill an already stressed-out city with incessant bell ringing, so I approved of them.

Especially when I kept hearing their voices behind me enthusiastically yelling out a list of what they were seeing:

"Yay, Santa!"

"Yay, Penguins!"

"... *Spandex!!*"

The bunnies' exclamations continued until they, too, passed me and Rebekah. And nothing reminds you that you run like a tortoise more than being passed by humans dressed as hares.

After that, I discovered one of my favorite racers of all: a guy playing Christmas carols on a tuba. He jogged while carrying that thing through the whole five-plus-mile race, slowing to walk and play songs every mile or so. When he played "We Three Kings" as the nativity set passed him, I decided I wanted to marry him. Thankfully, he was one of the few who never passed us, because I don't know if my ego would've recovered from bunnies, a human sleigh, *and* a tuba player all being faster than me.

Somewhere around mile four, the Nativity set pulled off to the side, apologetically announcing that "Baby Jesus is crying!" and so they ended up behind us, though not far behind. After they rejoined the race, they started singing carols, and that was another fun addition to the Christmas mayhem. In fact, I barely heard the jingle bells on all our shoes because there was so much else going on.

During the last mile, Rebekah looked around and proudly noted that we finally seemed to be passing quite a few people. I looked, too, and remarked that since we were passing people wrapped in Christmas tree lights, we really shouldn't let it go to our heads.

The ultimate point of that event was to have fun while running, and that we did.

> **PRO TIP:** If you're scared you'll be too slow to run a "serious" race, try a fun one first. Runners in those races are not pressured for time, and you'll probably meet a lot more people in your pace group who you can befriend and then maybe run a more serious race with in the future (if you're lucky, it may even be Tuba Guy).

Other things I have focused on for entertainment or to motivate me during races include:

- Fellow racers who sing along with their iPods. This can either be enjoyable, because of their lack of self-awareness and their joy of music, or it can be terrible and propel me to run faster to escape. Both are wins.

- Race fans' signs saying things like, "Run faster, my wife just passed gas!" Or, "Worst. Parade. Ever."

- Hearing people cheer for the one female who heads

into the bushes to pee with all the men.

- Continually passing perfect strangers who cheer me on or hand me marshmallows for an energy boost (that only happened once, but the strangers were a father and his little girl, and they were adorable).

- Slapping hands with people on the out-and-back stretches; especially people carrying a spare leg for their amputee husband who's running ahead of them. There's really nothing more motivating than that.

- Watching couples in front of me join hands during the last mile to spur each other to finish.

- Following a man wearing a shirt saying, "Death waits in the darkness" on the back, which is definitely motivating when you're trying not to pass out.

PRO TIP: Whether absurd or heart-string-tugging, there really are a lot of distractions in a race, and they can help you forget you're working out. Just hearing crowds along the course cheering and ringing cowbells for you can make you want to keep racing.

Another fun reward of races is that they give me the chance to catch up with my friends. I used the Army Ten-Miler a couple of years ago to reconnect with my friend

Laura. It worked, until she ran faster and left me behind. That turned out to be fine after all, because that race was full of other entertainment.

The Army Ten-Miler started and ended at the Pentagon. I began race day by struggling to find a place to park, which caused me to be late and flustered right from the beginning. I finally parked in a garage, exited my car, and stretched a tiny garbage bag around my upper torso because it was freezing outside, and that's a trick runners use to stay warm before a race. Except runners normally use bigger bags, which I didn't have, so I felt like an idiot. But I was a *warm* idiot, so I didn't care. I rushed down several floors to exit the garage, panicking and wearing a trash bag that trapped my arms inside. I looked like those people who play soccer with their torsos inside Zorb balls. (If you don't know what I'm talking about, search online right now for "Soccer in Zorb Balls" and watch whatever videos you find. You're welcome.)

Half woman, half garbage bag, I rushed to the start line. The bag was also Febreeze-scented, which added to the ridiculousness that was me at that point. I felt a tap on my shoulder and turned in surprise to see my friend Ryan, who immediately explained, "I saw this person rush past and I thought, *That trash bag is too small*, and it was you!" Typical. There were 30,000 people walking into that race, and someone I knew found me when I was wearing a scented straitjacket.

Ryan and I walked together to the start line and made

plans to do brunch after the race. (This leads me to yet another way to make racing fun: Promise your mouth French toast when it's over.) Then we separated (because he was in a faster corral than me, naturally). Finally warm enough, I removed my trash bag and began my quest to find Laura in a crowd of 30,000 runners. I called her on my phone and our conversation went something like this:

Me, staring into a sea of humanity: "Hey, I'm here!"

Her: "I'm right behind the purple arch of balloons! Wait... it's moving..."

Me, staring into the human sea while chasing an arch of moving purple balloons: "Okay... um... which side are you on? I'm now chasing the balloons."

Her: "Um... I'm kind of in the middle..."

Me: "Well, I'm over by the table with water. I'm *Jersey Shore* fist-pumping so you can see me." (Pumps fist like a frat boy on spring break.)

Her: "Oh! I know where that table is. Keep pumping! Keep pumping!"

I had replaced looking crazy in a tiny trash bag with looking crazy standing alone pumping my fist in the air, but it worked. Laura finally saw me.

We started the race together, but were only about two miles in before I could no longer keep up with her. Before we separated, we got to experience The Pee Bridge.

The name Pee Bridge refers to an area next to a bridge that has, through the years, become famous as the place in the Army Ten-Miler where males realize they need to pee and they do it there in solidarity. I've looked over and seen half a dozen men simultaneously using that area in plain view. Females tend to need a little more privacy, so we're typically forced to wait in the Porta-Potty lines instead.

After the Pee Bridge, I trotted along alone for a couple of miles and then surprisingly ran into another friend, Jose. We kept each other going by catching up on our love lives and our jobs until we crossed the finish line. (He may have also resorted to physically pulling me towards the finish line—multiple times—but it was mostly the conversation that kept me going.) Jose left and I headed to brunch, and that's when I realized the race organizers were only letting people exit the Pentagon one way—the long way—so our trek back to civilization started with an uphill climb, which was a sick joke to play on people who had just run ten miles.

A guy behind me made a comment about how cruel the hill was, and we started shuffling together. He was wearing an Army Ranger shirt and informed me that a) he had served in Mogadishu, and b) he was now old. I immediately liked him. He made it fun that we were trudging along with the masses like sheep. Every few steps he would announce something new:

"Everything south of my nipples hurts."

"In case anyone's wondering, there is no one who needs to pee right now more than I do."

"I'm just gonna say I did a half marathon today, since we're walking this far."

"They should have another water stop out here."

"If the Pentagon was a square, we would've turned by now... stupid place."

When we came up behind some other military guys, he announced to me, "I would start ragging on the other branches of the military, but I'm too tired to defend myself. I'd just let them beat me up for half an hour while saying, 'I'm sorry.'"

I felt sad to leave him.

Whether it's putting on a bunny costume and running with friends, or simply appreciating the whining coming out of the guy next to you, races offer moments when you can simply enjoy the people around you and feel happy. Unless you are a competitive runner at the front of the pack, in which case I assume that might feel kind of stressful. I doubt there are many bunnies up there.

MORAL OF THE STORY:

To keep your love of running fresh, sign up for races and then don't take yourself or anyone around you too seriously. Except that one woman going into the bushes to pee with the men—she means business.

Chapter 8

OTHER WAYS TO STAY MOTIVATED

» Tricks, Floss, and Zombies «

"The good Lord gave you a body that can stand most anything. It's your mind you have to convince."

VINCENT LOMBARDI

Even with all the positive things running has given me—better physical and mental health, satisfying friendships, stories that begin with introductions like, "*So there I was, running through electric wires ... again....*" I can't lie: I still have to use tricks to keep myself moving.

Sometimes I compete with myself, or think about what I've done in the past and how I can do that again and more. Sometimes I compete with the people around me. Like making sure I'm not the *first* one to lose consciousness in hot yoga class, or running up to pass someone on my regular running trail and yelling, "Kill!" (I don't actually do that, but mostly because I rarely find people I'm able to pass). Even if someone else is about to pass me, I still use that to push a little more. Whenever a boat started to pass us in a race, my rowing coach used to tell my team to "Make them work for it!" If you're about to pass me in a run, know that I may speed up like a jerk. Indulge me.

Sometimes I use cognitive theories to keep running, because I'm a nerd like that. There's a behavior change technique often used when someone asks us to sign a petition. Most of the time, a signature doesn't achieve anything directly. The bigger (sneakier?) purpose is cognitive. When I sign a petition to save the wombats, it signals my brain that I am someone who *does something* for the wombats. Then, when I'm approached again later and asked to do more—give money, host a wombat rally, whatever—I am more likely to do it, because I already took one step that proved to me that *I am a person who takes action for wombats.* If I don't take the next step, I'll feel like I'm betraying the person I am. So sometimes I will go for a run, even if I can only run for a few minutes, because just the simple act of getting out there signals to my brain that *I am a runner*: I am someone who runs. I am someone who runs and organizes peaceful protests for wombats. *That's who we are, brain. We just have to accept it.*

> **PRO TIP:** Fake it 'til you make it. Behave like a runner long enough and you eventually become one.

Visualization is another way I attempt to use my brain to manifest running success. Many athletes are trained to visualize their desired results—like crossing the finish line at their goal time—in order to subconsciously get their bodies to do what's necessary to achieve those results. I do that, too, except what I'm picturing is the Facebook status I'll post when I finish, and how cute my car will look wearing one of those 26.2 stickers marathoners buy to show they ran that many miles. I assume that's what Shalane Flanagan does, so I should be really fast soon using these methods.

Another trick I use to motivate myself to run is to "burn the ships." It's a reference my pastor used in a sermon. He was referring to a Spanish conquistador who, upon landing on some shore to start a conquest, ordered his men to burn their ships, leaving them no option to retreat. (I can't remember why my pastor was talking about Spanish conquistadors, and my church doesn't even own ships, but for some reason I was drawn to the idea of cutting off retreat options. Which seems pretty dramatic, now that I think of it, and I should probably figure out what he was talking about, in case he meant his staff would be blocking the exits the next time he gave a sermon.)

Anyway, back to burning the ships. Race fees are non-refundable, and bragging on social media about the race you are going to do is non-retractable. So sometimes I pay for races and announce them just to cut off my retreat routes until my heart catches up to my head in believing the race will be worth it. My head knows the race will be worth it—because they always are, and because there are always free bagels at the end–but my heart may need to be dragged along a bit before it agrees and stops attempting retreat.

> **PRO TIP:** Sign up for a race you have to get ready for. Don't overthink it, just lock yourself in before you lose your nerve. Now you and your heart have a reason to run more often until then, because there are dollars, pride, and bagels on the line.

Friends also offer motivation. Although I had the people in my marathon training program to encourage me during my race prep, my friends also helped get me to the finish line. Many helped raise money for my training program, others ran next to me when I needed company. Two friends actually tag-team-ran on the treadmill next to mine when ice on the road prevented me from logging the 13 miles I was supposed to do outside that day. If you've never experienced running 13 miles on a treadmill at a 5.5 mph pace, picture watching Lake Ontario filter through a Brita—only less exciting and more time consuming. Having people to talk to was a sanity saver.

Speaking of large quantities of liquid, that's another gift one of my friends gave me during marathon training. This was after I became dehydrated during my 18-miler and found myself face-down on my couch cushions, playing Russian Roulette with whether or not what was about to happen was another dry heave or more (me and running and vomit–the bond is real and it's deep). The ultimate friend offering was when, after my marathon was cut short in Nashville, a few friends offered to create an unofficial marathon in D.C. if I needed them to, just so I could finish one. Friends are huge motivators.

One way to find new friends is by joining running groups. My favorite group is a national veterans service organization called Team Red White and Blue. The team connects vets to their communities through a shared interest in physical activity. The support I've seen from everyone in this group has been beautiful. Some folks joined the group when they were near suicidal after combat experiences, and felt like they had no place in society. The group's warmth, combined with the health benefits from workouts, has literally saved people's lives. Sometimes when I'm struggling, I think of my friends from that group, their big hearts, and their "no one left behind" attitudes. Once when a couple of us admitted that we'd be slow in a race, one of the faster runners immediately jumped in and said, "If you guys are running that pace, then I'm running that pace." When a Team member weighing over 500 pounds started walking 5Ks to lose weight, dozens of other Team members rushed to the backs of races to walk with him. That group has honestly made me run more often, just so I can be around people like that.

> **PRO TIP:** Find your people. Whether you need people at your pace, or you just really want someone you can talk about cats with during a long run, they are out there somewhere. Start putting out feelers and they will come.

Another motivator I have for running comes from answering a classic question that I'm sure everyone asks when they're considering doing anything important in life, like choosing to become a surgeon or deciding to run for President: "What kind of outfits can I wear?" Clothing plays a surprisingly significant role in whether or not I feel motivated to run. Sometimes, I'll buy a new workout outfit and then run just to wear it. Other times, I'll change into running clothes even if I'm only considering a run, because I know the clothes will shame me into actually doing it. "Why are you wearing me if you aren't going to run?" my nylon shorts will ask. Obviously, then I have to hit the road just to shut those smug clothes up.

Sometimes I wear shirts with motivational mantras on them like "Never Quit." I read an article once about how repeating mantras like that can help if we find ourselves in a crisis. It focuses the mind and sustains the drive to keep fighting our way out of the situation. If I'm running when I'd rather be at brunch, that's basically the same as a crisis. If repeating the phrase on my shirt helps me finish faster, great. If chanting "I-never-quit" somehow morphs into "Eggs-Bene-dict" in my head, and that's actually what makes me finish faster, then so be it. Sometimes I'll wear the shirt of a group that I don't want to disappoint, like my Tough Mudder finisher shirt. Something about having everyone see that I got through a tough race or belong to a team makes it harder for me to get lazy and start walking–or whimpering–on the trail.

Clothing and accessories can be anti-motivators if used incorrectly, so one must inoculate oneself before a run. I get frustrated if my earbuds keep falling out or my shorts ride up because my thighs are fighting each other. And I assume a run in the rain would feel miserable if my long pants, say, got water-weighted and threatened to pull down enough to moon other runners, or my white shirt became translucent, or blood started dripping off my face (sure, the blood in question might turn out to be dye from the red baseball cap I chose to wear in pouring rain, but it could still be startling). I mean, I've *heard* those things can be miserable, if one were to make such obvious mistakes, which I don't. Anymore.

It definitely pays off to figure out what clothing and headphone choices work best. As for the thighs thing, that's probably here to stay—and that's why Body Glide exists. Because, Fashion Industry People, most women's thighs touch. Stop trying to make us think they don't.

Here's a non-exhaustive list of other tricks I use, in no particular order, to stay motivated with running:

Smiling. I've heard this sends a signal to the brain that whatever activity you are doing at that moment is enjoyable. At some points in a run, I'm willing to bray like a donkey if it'll make it seem more enjoyable, so yes, I've tried smiling.

Music. I download my favorite songs and then won't let myself listen to them unless I'm running. When I want to listen to one of the songs, I know I have to go for a run. This method is very scientific.

Other runners. Just when I hit the point where I want to scream like one of those goats in all those Internet videos, I'll pass another runner who gives me The Head Nod of

Approval, and then I feel like I can run another three miles.

Caffeine. Honestly, sometimes the only way I can get out there is to get some coffee in my system—otherwise, I continue to lie around somewhere in my apartment sleepy and angry. This is the same method I use when dealing with other humans in the morning: Let me drink my personality first, *then* you can safely approach me. If you use the coffee method of motivation, just don't drink too much before a really long run, because: bathrooms.

Gratitude. In all seriousness, sometimes thinking about people I've seen persevere, even though they're struggling more than I am in a race, or people who can't run at all, motivates me. I think of friends who have had accidents or who have heart disease and can't race. Or the wounded service members I've met who won't enjoy the sensation of running with both legs again. I've seen guys take off their prosthetic legs and jump into wheelchairs to play basketball, and I saw a woman who'd been paralyzed in a training accident go on to play sled hockey for Team USA. These are people who choose to focus not on asking, "Why me?" Instead, they ask, "Ok, what are the new possibilities?" When I'm struggling to get through a run, I think of them and what a privilege it is to be able to run with my body, just as it is. And then I run harder, because I feel like I owe it to those people to do so.

Skinny jeans. As cliché as it is, getting thinner and more toned is still a motivator for me to run. Whether it's about looking hot in front of an ex, or making sure I don't have too much face on my face bones, I know running plays a role in my ability to feel cute and fit in my wardrobe. (The face bones phrase came from a conversation between two of my friends where one told the other that she had "nice face bones," to which the other responded, "Yeah. I just have too much … face on them." Whenever I gain weight, I can see it in the amount of excess face I have on my face bones, and I know I need to run more.)

Injuries. The older I get, the more I realize that if I'm not consistent and don't train enough, I risk straining, pulling, or stress-fracturing something the next time I do decide to run. I'm still not great at that aspect of running, but I'm trying. Not being great at that is how I ended up lying on a table, staring at the ceiling trying not to giggle as I isolated the muscles in my buttocks at the command of a physical therapist, instead of running like I intended to do that day. My knee had swelled, causing me to find out that I had alignment issues I needed to work on and that I needed to train more consistently if I wanted to keep doing endurance challenges. I went on to experience "dry needling" in order to improve knee function, which basically includes having little needles, at times zapped with electric pulses, probe various muscles. So, really, electricity, running, and I might actually have a closer relationship than vomiting, running, and I enjoy. Either way, I think running and I need to get some new friends.

Zombies. I haven't personally used this motivator (yet), but there's apparently an app that helps runners perform interval training (alternating sprinting and slowing down throughout an entire run, which helps increase speed) by telling you how close zombies are to your back and making you run away from them in spurts. I usually do a version of this by picking out a target in the distance, like a lamp post (and by "lamp post" I mean "shirtless runner"), and sprinting until I reach it, then slowing down again. But running from zombies sounds fun, too.

And, lastly…

Floss. I don't know why, but for some reason I started finding disposable floss sticks *everywhere*, including during my runs. When I started mentioning it, I caused my friends all over the country to start seeing them more too. So now there's this weird, dental-hygienicky connection between us all, because we tell each other when we see them and they make everyone think of me. I wish I knew how to harness this gift and redirect it so that I found $100 bills instead. I suppose it could be worse, like if I kept seeing hippos, and then those reminded everyone of me. In any case, I sometimes distract myself by looking for floss sticks on my runs.

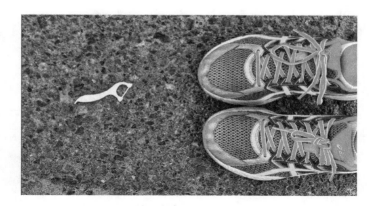

Apparently, there's a part of our brains called the reticular activating system that causes us to start noticing things more after we first become aware of them, like when we see other cars like the one we drive, or when we hear the same ring tone as our own on other people's cell phones. So it makes sense that I see more of these dental hygiene things now that I've become more aware of them, but it still begs the question: Why are so many people flossing in public, and why are they dropping the sticks all willy-nilly afterwards?

If all of my motivation tricks fail, I can also distract myself by simply looking around. The light hits objects and bathes them in different colors, depending on the time of day, or the weather, or the season. Maybe I see a tree that's starting to bloom, or some snow that hasn't given up yet. I've even noticed one lone daffodil growing proudly by itself, away from the cluster of other daffodils nearby, and was moved by the symbolism of that whole

"Bloom where you're planted" saying. I got emotional, but since I saw that lone daffodil near the end of my run, I could've been emotional simply because I knew I could soon put on guilt-free sweat pants and wear them for the rest of the day. In any case, running is a good excuse to get outside and look around.

> **PRO TIP:** Running outside allows us to experience the real world briefly before we go back to looking at it only though Instagram posts on our computers.

Sometimes motivation comes in waves, and you just have to ride out the times when it's not happening so much. To illustrate how this works, here's a chronological look at my motivation levels on a typical run:

- Beyonce starts to sing to me and I begin my run.

- I pass a man on a bike who leers at me, and I make a face and run faster.

- I immediately slow down again, because I'm only a half-mile in and I already want to stop.

- I check to see how fast I'm running and then get angry and sad.

- *Oh, thank goodness.* I've at least done one mile. I wonder if I can take a walk break now.

- "Harlem Shake" comes on my playlist, and I have to resist the urge to stop and do the Bernie dance.

- I adjust my shorts.

- I adjust my arm band.

- I pass a ridiculously ripped girl wearing only a sports bra and a pair of shorts she clearly stole from a 4-year-old.

- I smile. She doesn't. I hate her and want to be her, simultaneously.

- Around this point, on various runs, I've seen a man nearly drive into the river, a man walking his giant pet snake, and a lady Rollerblading with a cocker spaniel on her shoulders. This is not far from the general area where I once tripped over nothing and skinned my leg from knee to ankle. I remain on high alert in this area.

- I adjust my shorts.

- I adjust my arm band.

- I hit the place where I try to look like a good runner because people in cars can see me as they drive past.

- I come to the area where people in cars can no longer see me and I resume the pace of a one-year-old climbing stairs.

- I'm so tired that when I pass another runner, the only

thing I can do in acknowledgement is nod almost imperceptibly.

- Another runner passes me and bares his teeth like a Doberman. *Yes sir, I understand you are attempting to smile and physically can't right now. I see your grimace, and raise you an eye blink substitute for a head nod, in acknowledgement of your existence.*

- I make an audible grunting noise in protest of this whole running thing.

- I freeze and glance around, wondering how loud that grunt was, since I'm wearing headphones.

- I lose all sense of pride and start to bob my head and mouth the words to a Kanye West song to distract me from running.

- I adjust my shorts.

- I adjust my arm band.

- I finally hit a place where I'm close enough to my house that I'll let myself walk shame-free the rest of the way.

- A cute runner passes me and I try to lie to him with my eyes, like *Yeah, I just finished my run and I was super-fast and awesome at it too, so we are kindred running spirits and should probably date each other.* I am able to move my face muscles to actually smile at him. He looks effortlessly swift and makes me wonder why

I even try to run.

- I finally get back to my house, sweaty, and dejected, but then Olympic Gold Medalist Sonya Richards-Ross tells me through my running app that I did a good job. So, naturally, I immediately start planning my run for the next day.

If all else fails, I watch Jerry Dobson's *Welcome to the Grind* sports motivational video on YouTube. If that doesn't fire you up, you're probably not breathing and have bigger issues than trying to make yourself run.

....

MORAL OF THE STORY:

Not everyone is motivated by *Runner's World* covers. Find your own floss stick or chatty running shorts and use them to fuel your own runs.

Chapter 9

THE REWARDS
» Finger Traps and Free Therapy «

"If you don't have answers to your problems after a four-hour run, you ain't getting them."

CHRISTOPHER MCDOUGALL, BORN TO RUN

So why do I keep pushing myself in a sport that doesn't come naturally for me?

The crazy adventures I've had in training and racing definitely keep me coming back for more. Whenever I start feeling lazy, or like I don't want to do another challenge, I remember how great I felt after the last one. Plus, sometimes you just want to wear an accessory made of ribbon and pewter—and getting a race medal is really the best way I've found to satisfy that craving.

But there are many more reasons besides the memory of past fun and the post-race heavy necklaces that keep me in a long-term relationship with running. Some reasons are communal. I meet new friends and get inspired by others. Other reasons are personal. Running has become a companion to me. It's always there when I want it, and it helps me become a better version of myself through the lessons I learn by doing it. Here's a summary of the major benefits I've gained from running:

Free Therapy

I've processed friend drama and heartbreak on the running trail. I've grappled with decisions and returned from runs with more clarity. I've thought through situations I felt I handled poorly, and run until I got to the root of the issue. I've laughed. I've cried. I've talked to God during runs—like that day I was dealing with an extremely uncomfortable situation with someone at work, and prayed for help to let go of the stress on my run. A few minutes later, I found myself performing a series of deer-in-the-headlights movements, completely forgetting about work as I laid terrified eyes on a five-foot-long snake wrapped around the shoulders of someone standing next to the running path. *Dear Lord, that wasn't what I meant when I asked for help forgetting about today, but, hey—works for me.*

Running helps me manage overwhelming emotions. There's something about the movement that's calming. Being in motion distracts me enough to make me lift my mental gaze off whatever I'm obsessing about, and gives me just enough of a break to let some calmness seep in. It's like the adult form of being rocked to sleep, without actually having to go to sleep and without the awkwardness I assume would accompany asking another adult to hold me on their lap.

I read an article once that said the act of making simple decisions aids in getting ourselves back on track when we feel overwhelmed. Sometimes I feel paralyzed by the amount of work I need to do, or by the number of options in the shampoo section at Target. Why do we have to face this kind of stress? So I run. Because running doesn't require me to think much. It gives me one discreet task to accomplish. Accomplishing that one thing frees up my head and heart to deal with all the other things, like making the difficult decision to sentence my hair to moisture and shine versus sleekness and bounce.

Resilience

I've tripped and fallen during runs, but then gotten back up, which showed me how to be resilient about other things in life. Running has taught me that I can persevere. I remember struggling through a break-up once and a friend spurred me on with, "You ran a marathon! You can get through *this*!" It made me smile, because she was right. Running is symbolic. It shows me that I'm the type of person who can overcome things, even when I'm downright miserable. The silly signs of encouragement that people hold up during races start to work their way into my psyche and I think, *Yes, my feet* are *hurting, because I* am *kicking so much butt! That sign is correct!*

Discipline

I've learned that when I'm disciplined in one area, like running, it spills over into the rest of my life. When I start my day by working out, I find myself making better eating choices throughout the day, or leaving my apartment a little tidier. I'm a more squared-away version of myself—maybe not completely responsible and adult-shaped, but markedly less train-wrecky.

Confidence

So many times, I've thought a race was too exclusive or too difficult for someone like me to finish, but after I completed those races and discovered that I had what it took to finish them, it made me braver about trying other things in my life. Like maybe I *could* go on a jungle safari, or get my master's degree, or survive a grocery store unarmed after the weatherman has predicted a blizzard.

> **PRO TIP:** Running makes you feel fierce. Be prepared to strut when you return from a run. Or, depending on how sore you are, at least be prepared to waddle with attitude.

The Chance to Prove Myself

When I push through more miles on a run than ever before, I reach a deeper conviction about what I'm made of. When I run in nasty weather instead of staying inside wearing furry slippers, I get to feel like a superhero. (When some guy saw me heading out for a run in the rain, I said, "I actually like the rain," to which he replied, "Yeah, because running in the rain makes you feel like a superhero!" Before he said that, I was going to say that the rain keeps me cooled off... but, sure, let's go with his reason.) Sometimes it's hard to find chances to prove ourselves in modern daily life. Creating a really compelling PowerPoint presentation is rewarding and all, but it's not the same as physically pushing ourselves and fighting for something.

Cheering fans don't fill stadiums to watch someone reconcile expense accounts. They come to watch people play sports. Granted, winning a game or crossing a finish line isn't the same as curing cancer, but I think we love it anyway because it's symbolic. Something inside of us needs to see people physically fight for something. Even better, we need to fight for something ourselves. We're wired with a desire to strive and exert force and use our muscles and compete—and lose and learn and battle again, with more humility and more wisdom. It fills a void inside us that working only our brains in cushy, air-conditioned buildings can't. It feeds the inner caveman part of our souls that wants to yell things like, "I have made *fire!*"

Raw Simplicity

In a society where we move ourselves from place to place in everything from cars to planes to those odd-looking Segway things that *no one* looks desirable on, there's something satisfying and liberating about covering ground solely by moving our own bodies. Plus, if you live in D.C., where parking is a blood sport, running is even more attractive. There are many more spots open to park a body than a car.

Increased Mental Toughness

I can get extremely frustrated by how quickly my fitness level drops if I start skipping runs. When that happens, I feel like I'm starting all over again to build up endurance and bring my speed back up. I can get discouraged and consider running to be too much effort... or I can allow it to change me. I can view running as a metaphor for life and let it teach me how to keep going when I hit setbacks.

I've found that if I decide I'm only going to run two miles, I'll struggle at the end of those two miles, but if I decide to run four miles, I won't start struggling until I get close to the fourth mile. This tells me I sometimes hold back, and that I'm often capable of more. It helps me employ more mental grit during my runs. It probably also means I'm capable of using that grit to resist the siren song of anything made of dark chocolate or goat cheese, but let's not get ahead of ourselves.

> **PRO TIP:** So much of running is a mental game. But so is so much of life, so why not get out on the trail and push against all the *No* that lives inside us? Then there won't be so much *No* left when we want to try other things, like moving to that dream city and starting over, or finally applying for that job as a baby-tiger nanny. (Note: I have never actually heard of that job but if it exists, I need to know. *Because I would rock that job.*)

Patience

It always feels like a struggle in the early parts of my runs, before my body settles into the rhythm. I have to remind myself it will get better around the one-mile mark, because it always does. This teaches me patience, which I can tap into at other times, like when I meet a new group of people. I can remind myself it takes a while to form bonds. Not everyone likes having someone excitedly jump on them like a beagle when they're first introduced. I can use some of that patience I've learned in running and give it a minute.

Knowing How to Relax

As a Type A personality, I can be hard on myself. I may get obsessive about a goal and fight the process of getting there more than I need to. Running has given me Chinese finger trap lessons. A finger trap is a tube made of woven material. If you stick one index finger in each end, the way the material is woven makes it so that if you try to pull your fingers out, the tube grips to trap them inside. The more you struggle, the worse it gets. The key to freeing your fingers is to relax and actually push in a little, counter-intuitively. One day, when I was desperately trying to run faster than normal, I breathlessly looked down at my watch to check my pace and realized I was running slower than normal. I got so mad I stopped trying altogether and ended my run in disappointment and frustration. The next day, I gave up worrying about my pace and just ran for the joy of movement, doing the opposite of what I thought it would take to improve my speed. At the end of the run, I discovered my pace had increased. Good one, finger trap!

Befriending Failure

When I don't achieve the pace I want or I can't finish a distance, I gain something really important: I learn that failure won't kill me. Failing is an important part of growing. We've all seen or heard of the adult who grew up never being told No, the guy who was always given an honorary home run in tee-ball. That guy is typically not particularly enjoyable to be around, and that never-hearing-a-no mentality is going to be pretty debilitating for him sooner or later. Life can't be absolutely controlled, so if we aren't familiar with struggle, we tend to panic and crumble when it finally finds us. Whereas, if we've gone through something tough, like failure, we will fear it less when we approach it again. I try to go into a run comfortable with the idea that I may face disappointment. By keeping my expectations flexible, I can appreciate whatever the run brings, even if it's a lesson in failure.

> **PRO TIP:** Running can be a lab environment to test all kinds of things in ourselves, including patience, perseverance, and the ability to not throw your sneakers at someone when you fail. Results may vary.

Helping Others

In addition to all the personal rewards, running has taught me how great it feels to help others persevere. One morning when I was at a gym, slogging through the miles during marathon training, the lady on the treadmill next to me said, "I was going to stop, but then you kept going and it inspired me to keep going!" That, of course, made me want to keep going even more. It's a wonder she and I aren't still on those treadmills, continuing like two high school kids trying to end a phone conversation: "*You* get off the treadmill first!" "No *you*!" "No *you*!"

Another time, I ended up running next to a woman during a race, and she was going a little slower than I was. I could've gone ahead or not taken so many walk breaks, but I felt like I should stay with her instead. When we crossed the finish line, I found out that was the fastest time she'd ever logged at that distance. She told me I was the one who helped her keep going. Seeing how excited she was and being part of her success was way more rewarding than running the race just for myself. Plus, the slower you run, the better your race photos look, because you're not all grimacing and scrunched up from the effort, so I totally nailed those race photos.

Running gives us the space to cheer for each other. I pass strangers on every run who give a little wave or yell out support. There is solidarity in the running community, and that includes support beyond just the running. When you encourage someone on the trail or at the finish line, you're also encouraging them in life in general.

I once watched a Paralympics-type competitive event. One of the last track events was a wheelchair race. As the racers made their way around the track, I watched two of the men fall way behind everyone else, obviously struggling. Then I realized only one was struggling—the other was sacrificing his own race to stay and help. That single moment bolstered my hope for the human race. Granted, it also made me come dangerously close to dissolving into an Ugly Cry, but it was worth it.

We may not see the people we cheer for or run next to in a race, ever again. We aren't likely to be there to encourage them in their marriages or their careers. But for this one time–for these few minutes–we can scream our hearts out for them and help them go further. We aren't only cheering for them in the race, we're pushing our encouragement into them for whatever they might be facing next.

The Benefits Keep on Coming

Running offers so many inspirational moments. I'm inspired when I see the sculpted bodies in the front of the pack glide effortlessly away from me at the start of a race (so quickly they glide away from me, so very quickly). Even more, I'm inspired when I see the people who struggle. And I'm not alone. I've heard stories of really fast competitive runners saying they're in awe of us back-of-the-packers, and for multiple reasons. One competitive runner once marveled at a slower man in my running group. The faster man was so used to finishing races in a relatively short amount of time that he hadn't really realized how much longer slower runners have to keep their bodies in motion in order to finish. Amazed, he blurted out, "How can you keep running for *that long*?" We slower runners may not get points for speed, but you gotta give us points for perseverance.

I read a story recently, written by a serious runner, in which he admitted that he wouldn't run if it didn't come so naturally. He said the people who run when it doesn't come easily are the ones who inspire him.

I have to agree. The people who are substantially over-weight, who really struggle to finish, who run for a loved one, who are blind and run next to a guide, who have a prosthesis—they send a powerful message. They are in-your-face reminders that we all have the capability inside us to overcome so much.

> **PRO TIP:** If you run long enough, you'll come across really inspiring people. Sometimes you'll even discover that you're one of them for someone else—especially if you're struggling. So don't let the fear of struggling through a race keep you from doing it. You may be just the inspiration someone else needs.

Being inspired by others has definitely helped me finish races, like The Xterra 10K Trail Run I did several years ago in Richmond, Virginia. I started the race with my friend Sarah, but she quickly left me behind (more precisely, I was so much slower than her that she took a nasty spill, pulled a hamstring, fell in poison ivy, suffered a deep cut to her knee, and I didn't see any of it. Then she still finished before me.)

I was ok with Sarah leaving me, because I somehow got mixed in with a group of runners dedicated to raising funds and awareness for wounded veterans by participating in extreme feats of physical endurance. The team included members who had lost limbs in combat but still ran. The group members always wore gas-masks during races, to add to their extremeness. Even without seeing their faces through the masks, I thought they were dreamy.

As we all lined up at the starting line, Sarah joked that if she passed the masked guys during the race, she was going to pinch their butts. I guess my pace was what a really in-shape person would run if their breathing was restricted, because I got tangled up in their little gas-masked formation. Two of them passed me by, breathing like Darth Vader, and then a third put his hand on my back and gestured for me to get in front of him on the path. Naturally, since I was passing him, I considered pinching his butt, but instead I got all worried I was in their way and stammered, "I'm sorry!" as I fell in line. Eventually they all passed me, but I stayed not too far behind them. Whenever I felt tired, it was nice to look up and see them being all strong, consistent, supportive. Did

I mention strong? They were a nice distraction, indeed.

I continued along all the obstacles in the trail run—through rivers, across boulders, up hills—without incident. That is, until I got to the last bridge, about a mile from the finish line. Halfway across the bridge, I suddenly felt nauseous–like, hanging-over-the-side-of-the-bridge-and-heaving nauseous. (Seriously, how many times can one person vomit during races in their lifetime before some kind of mercy rule kicks in?) The nausea came out of nowhere and shocked me. I'd take a few steps and then have to bend over the railing again. The whole episode lasted so long I'm sure I gave other runners a great story to share at the end: "Did you see that girl heaving over the bridge? I heard that her friend was run over by a bus and *still* finished before her." I finally felt better and started jogging again, and soon saw the gas-mask guys up ahead. I decided I wanted to finish with them, so I jogged faster.

When I fell in behind the guys, I settled into their cadence. It was fun to be near them because everyone along the route started cheering wildly for what they were doing, which was great, until they stopped in the race's exit chutes for photo-taking and handshaking and whatnot. I was stuck behind them, so my stomach thought it would be hilarious to feel nauseous again when I had no escape—*and* an audience. There may be great photos somewhere of an awesome team of guys in gas-masks... and the girl behind them losing her Gatorade.

(You might think that was the most embarrassing thing that happened in regard to that race, but you'd be wrong. Later, when I wrote about the race on my blog—including about my affection for the gas-mask men—one of them saw it and contacted me to give me more information about their organization. He made a joke that he was glad I didn't actually pinch his butt. And he was actually a *she*. Apparently, there was one female runner under those masks. Sometimes things happen that make you wish you were *only* vomiting in public.)

Situations like heaving at the finish line prove that running can definitely be humbling. But running also offers a sense of pride. It feels undeniably good to get out there when you know so many people choose not to— and one of those people may even be your former self. When you get out and run, you are now someone who *does* things, who is powerful.

I remember reading the bio the Navy put out for me when I first joined. Somewhere in it was the phrase "accomplished athlete." I laughed when I first read that, because I thought it was a gross overstatement and made me sound like I'd really done something. Then I took inventory of the races I'd completed over the years, some of which I had mentioned during the Navy application process, and I realized–I *did* sound like an accomplished athlete. When did *that* happen?

MORAL OF THE STORY:

Although you may not be the fastest or even the most dedicated person, running will embrace you anyway and offer you rewards beyond your expectation. One day, you won't even recognize yourself, not with all those medals, all that patience, and all those stories of tossing your cookies. And it'll be awesome.

Chapter 10

STILL A STRUGGLE
» My Future as a Runner «

"My sweatpants smell like give up."

UNKNOWN

Even after all these years and all the great adventures I've had, I'll admit it's still a struggle to keep running.

Some days I can't do it. Running imitates life, and sometimes I dig around and can't unearth enough willpower to get out on the trail, just like some days I can't summon the determination to stop eating spoonfuls of Nutella, or can't keep from honking when someone willfully ignores the one-in-one-out zipper method rule of interstate vehicle merging (which is obviously how anarchy begins). We all have our breaking points.

In addition to struggling with willpower, I also still struggle to call myself a "real" runner. Mostly because I'm not fast, but also because I'm not some crazy, super-dedicated mile-logger. Honestly, I typically do the least amount of training I feel I can get away with in order to still be able to finish the races I want to do. Kind of like I did the least amount of piano practice in order to pull off my recitals as a kid. You heard me, Mrs. Roland. I'm not proud to admit it, but a seven-year-old has other priorities.

I also sometimes still get scared to run with other people. Maybe it's because of that one time when I started a military running test with the Navy and finished with the Army, because the depth of my slowness outlasted an entire branch of the U.S. Armed Forces. I began seeing a totally different uniform pass me before I finally completed the test. The Army had been waiting to do their running test on the track the Navy was using and they finally got tired of waiting for me to finish and released their soldiers anyway. When I later told that story to my friend Rebecca, she looked at me with a mixture of amusement and pity, as if looking at a pet fighting a part of its own body. "You really have a lot of heart!" she finally blurted out, which I assume was code for, "I didn't realize anyone could be that bad at something and want to keep doing it in public anyway!" I suppose that would be enough to humble any mammal with the capacity for self-awareness.

> **PRO TIP:** Feel free to re-read the story above whenever you feel like you can't finish a race. If I'm that slow and I can still finish endurance challenges without being swept off the course, you must now believe you can too.

I get anxious about running with others because I sometimes still feel like an imposter waiting to be uncovered. Even after having countless races under my belt, along with medals and headbands proclaiming I've conquered endurance challenges most Americans haven't, I still sometimes feel like I'm not *really* in the runners club. I'll see someone wearing a marathon shirt and, even though I have also finished a marathon, a tiny voice inside will say, *Yeah, but you only did* one. *And you walked at times. And it took you longer than Oprah to finish, so let's not get carried away.*

I've learned to push those doubts aside. When I start to

feel sorry for myself or start to get aggravated during a run, I think of something my friend Gina's cross country coach used to tell her during practices in the rain: "It's raining on everyone." That's such a great, simple reminder to shuck the victim mentality and stop feeling sorry for myself. Yeah, I'm slow and running can be hard. But life can be hard. For anyone. *So get over it and get this done.* I don't want to be someone who only *thought* about doing a race. Only *considering* pushing myself doesn't feel like enough. It's when I *actually* push myself that I can look myself in the eye with respect.

Do I think running will always be a struggle for me? I do. I expect to always feel the urge to pre-apologize to other runners for being slow.

I expect to always start to add a "but" caveat after I utter the phrase "I'm a runner," to let people know that although I've logged hundreds of miles, my lack of consistency and lack of speed may make me, in their eyes, not a "real" runner. I'm keenly aware of that.

I expect to begrudgingly start runs when I'd rather be at home in furry slippers.

I expect days when my legs feel like they weigh 200 pounds each and a scream goes off in my brain imploring me to go back to the couch.

But I also expect more head nods and waves along the way, more inspiring moments, and more free therapy during stretches of time when there's only me and the pavement. I expect more times when I get stressed and a friend reminds me that what I probably need to do is go for a run.

And I *will* run. Because, even with all the doubts and struggles, I am a runner. And that is what we runners do. We run.

Occasionally we wear tutus and get electrocuted, but mostly we run.

....

MORAL OF THE STORY:

You can be a runner, too. (And you don't even have to put on a tutu or get electrocuted. Unless you want to.)

Contact me at *DCDana.com* to share your own running adventures. I'd love to hear them!

Acknowledgments

Thank you to everyone who has run beside me in races and in life. To so many who helped during this process and with my running through the years (Cherilyn Crowe, Gina Gray, Gina Junio, John Papa, Alicia Long, Kami Swingle, Heather(s) and Matt(s) (Ryersons and Carlsons), Jill Wyman, Stacie Davis, Laura Kanzler, Sadrian (Sarah Leslie and Adrian Schulte), the Lee Besties, Robin Camarote, Angela Lauria and the other members of the Difference Press family, Sean Wolridge, Rebecca Johnson, Rebekah Krimmel, Adam Knapp, My DC Tribe, and so many others).

Thank you to Team in Training for making me a marathoner; to Brian Wright, Susie Nguyen, Dan Ohlstein, and others for making me a Tough Mudder; for Team Red White and Blue for continuing to feed my addiction; and to my Ragnar and Run Now Relay teams. Thank you to God for the ability to enjoy running, and for talking to me during runs, even if through terrifying snakes.

And, finally, thank you to my parents, for unconditional love, support, and for trying to suppress their fear and disbelief whenever I mention the strange race I want to run next.

About the Author

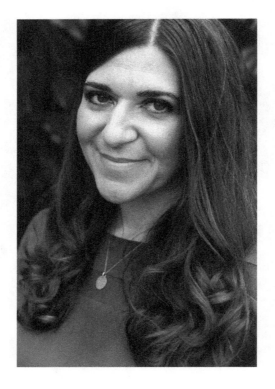

Dana accidentally became a runner more than 10 years ago and has logged a vast array of average finish times since. Her running accomplishments include completing dozens of races and obstacle courses, a full marathon, a Tough Mudder, and multi-day relay events involving little sleep and smelly vans. Dana has proven it's possible to be a long-term runner without gaining much speed, losing much weight, or sacrificing a fairly lax approach to exercise.

Dana started her career as a White House staffer and currently works for a large management consulting firm in Washington, D.C. A mix of serendipity and Murphy's Law typically accompanies her running, travel, and love-life adventures. This combination has landed her everywhere—from living on a bluegrass band's tour bus, to supporting disaster response activities, to being electrocuted while naked in a Japanese bath house. She writes about all of it on her humor blog, DCDana.com.

Dana holds a master's degree in communication and serves as a Public Affairs Officer for the U.S. Navy Reserve. Her writing has appeared in local newspapers, online magazines, and in particularly enthralling government PowerPoint presentations.

Dana currently resides in Arlington, Virginia. In addition to running, her hobbies include seeking out reasons to wear a tutu and finding floss on her running trail.